THE
AYURVEDIC
RESET DIET

"Vatsala Sperling has gathered a lifetime of cultural influence, serious study, and daily practice into this book. I have sat at Vatsala's table and eaten her food. She knows how to create a life-affirming, healthy, peaceful oasis and offers wisdom and guidance on how to accomplish exactly that. Ayurveda means 'science of life.' In this remarkably thorough work, Vatsala provides all the knowledge required to bring life into your kitchen and your home. This is beautiful stuff."

CHRISTOPHER S. KILHAM, AUTHOR OF
THE FIVE TIBETANS AND *THE WHOLE FOOD BIBLE*

"In *Ayurvedic Reset Diet* Vatsala Sperling presents practical tools and authentic Ayurvedic guidance with precision and insight. The book is replete with practical methods that one can integrate into everyday life with ease to achieve better health and wellness."

SHUBHRAJI, FOUNDER OF NAMAH VEDANTA CENTER
AND AUTHOR OF *IN THE LOTUS OF THE HEART*

"*The Ayurvedic Reset Diet* is an easy-to-read guide to using basic Ayurvedic principles to achieve health. Most people, especially in the West, have been conditioned to eating in ways that actually rob them of vibrant health and often lead to illness. This book offers a way out of that routine. Vatsala explains very clearly how and why to follow simple dietary guidelines to recover health in a very down-to-earth way. By explaining the rationale for the guidelines, the author makes it even easier to apply them. This is one of those books that can make a big difference for anyone motivated to achieve better health. I recommend it highly."

ALAN V. SCHMUKLER, CHIEF EDITOR OF
HOMEOPATHY 4 EVERYONE

"I have met many doctors—allopathic, Ayurvedic, and naturopathic—and the best have one thing in common: they were raised by healers. They grew up in a living tradition, imbibing everyday wisdom from a parent or grandparent. Vatsala falls into this category and seamlessly combines her medical knowledge with traditional know-how. For those of us who didn't have the good fortune to be raised in such an environment, this book provides the next best thing."

SIMON CHOKOISKY, AUTHOR OF
THE FIVE DHARMA TYPES

OTHER WORKS BY VATSALA SPERLING
from the Heart of the Indian Tradition

*Classic Tales from India: How Ganesh Got His Elephant Head
and Other Stories*

Arjuna: The Gentle Warrior

*The Magical Adventures of Krishna: How a Mischief Maker
Saved the World*

Ganga: The River That Flows from Heaven to Earth

Karna: The Greatest Archer in the World

Hanuman's Journey to the Medicine Mountain

Ram the Demon Slayer

How Parvati Won the Heart of Shiva

How Ganesh Got His Elephant Head

*For Seven Lifetimes: An East-West Journey
to a Spiritually Fulfilling and Sustainable Marriage*
(coauthor Ehud Sperling)

THE
AYURVEDIC
RESET DIET

Radiant Health through Fasting, Mono-Diet, and Smart Food Combining

Vatsala Sperling, MS, Ph.D., PDHom, CCH, RSHom

Healing Arts Press
Rochester, Vermont

Healing Arts Press
One Park Street
Rochester, Vermont 05767
www.HealingArtsPress.com

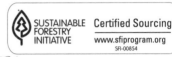

Text stock is SFI certified

Healing Arts Press is a division of Inner Traditions International

*Note to the reader: This book is intended as an informational guide. The remedies,
approaches, and techniques described herein are meant to supplement, and not to be a
substitute for, professional medical care or treatment. They should not be used to treat
a serious ailment without prior consultation with a qualified health care professional.*

Cataloging-in-Publication Data for this title is available from the Library of Congress

ISBN 978-1-64411-130-7 (print)
ISBN 978-1-64411-131-4 (ebook)

Printed and bound in the United States by Lake Book Manufacturing, Inc.
The text stock is SFI certified. The Sustainable Forestry Initiative® program
promotes sustainable forest management.

10 9 8 7 6 5 4 3 2 1

Text design by Debbie Glogover and layout by Virginia Scott Bowman
This book was typeset in Garamond Premier Pro, Gill Sans, and Legacy Sans with
Jazmin and Kapra Neue Pro used as display typefaces

To send correspondence to the author of this book, mail a first-class letter to the
author c/o Inner Traditions • Bear & Company, One Park Street, Rochester, VT
05767, and we will forward the communication, or contact the author directly at
www.rochesterhomeopathy.com.

Contents

Acknowledgments

The foundation for this book was laid decades ago, when I was just a little girl and a very ardent student eager to learn everything my mother could teach me by way of being a living example. If mothers are considered our first teachers, I was very lucky to get a fantastic one. She knew the art of living and the science of life as explained in Ayurveda, Homeopathy, and the ancient culture of India, and she taught with love. To this mother, I will be forever and always grateful.

My gratitude also flows in the direction of my father, Shri Ramnath, my brother Shri Bala Subramaniam, and my dear sisters, Meenakshi, Rajalakshmi, Bhuvaneshwari, and Vijayalakshmi. Each one of them has shown me the way to live with love and respect for nature.

My in-laws, Helen and Julius Sperling, were always charmed by my activities in the kitchen, and my father-in-law found many parallels between the Jewish kosher laws and the science of food preparation based on Ayurveda. My sister- and brother-in-law, Debora and Bob Kanig, both die-hard devotees of everything organic, natural, and sustainable, filled me with enthusiasm for the subject of organic foods in the United States, and I was happy to recall that I was raised on seasonal homegrown, cooked-from-scratch organic foods, way before the word *organic* became fashionable in the United States.

My background in Ayurveda comes not from a college degree in the subject but from having watched my family and even my neighbors live their lives according to the principles laid out in Ayurveda. To these individuals, I will be grateful always.

How I became a homeopath is a different story altogether, and for it, I am forever in debt to my dear husband, Ehud C. Sperling. His love of learning, his curiosity, and his relentless striving to keep his family in the fold of alternative medicine and an unconventional lifestyle propelled me toward an education in Homeopathy. His lifelong passion for exploring and understanding other cultures and other ways of being infected me too and led me to study the life of our hunter-gatherer ancestors and explore the possibility of integrating Ayurvedic principles into my practice of Homeopathy.

Our son, Mahar, has been asking "Why?" ever since he began speaking, and in order to give him correct answers on Ayurvedic food rules, I had to do research and educate myself on the facts. He keeps me on my toes and for that I am grateful.

My thanks are due to my dear friend Leslie Blair. She has unconditionally loved and supported me through every adventure in my life, be it Ayurvedic vegetarian cooking, writing, or practicing Homeopathy.

My thanks are due also to Isabel and Vilma Solano Rojas. Their selfless and devoted service has enabled me to follow my heart without a care in the world and avail myself of extended periods of time, which I could devote to research and writing.

I am very happy to have the great opportunity to be published by Inner Traditions, Ehud's book publishing company. The former chairman of Tata Steel, J. R. D. Tata, once said, "A company is only as great as the people who work in it." If this is indeed the yardstick for measuring a great company, then I am delighted to say that the people at Inner Traditions, from those at the front desk to those in the corner office, are some of the best in the industry. It is my pleasure and honor to have them publish my book.

Finally, my gratitude and heartfelt thanks are due to Swamiji Bhoomananda Tirtha, my guru since I was five years old. On occasions when I was stuck and needed assistance, he helped me with no strings attached. Without his timely support, I do not know what I would have done. Swamiji, I am forever grateful to you.

VATSALA SPERLING, MS, PH.D., PDHOM, CCH, RSHOM

अन्नपूर्णे सदापूर्णेशङ्करप्राणवल्लभे |
ज्ञानवैराग्यसिद्ध्यर्थं भिक्षां देहि च पार्वति ||11||

Annapuurnne Sadaa-Puurnne Shangkara-Praanna-Vallabhe |
Jnyaana-Vairaagya-Siddhyartham Bhikhssaam Dehi Cha Paarvati ||

O Mother Anna Poorna, you, who is always full of gift of
food and blessings, you, who is the the beloved of Shankara;

O Mother Parvati, please grant me the alms of your grace,
for awakening within me spiritual knowledge and freedom
from all worldly desires.

माता च पार्वती देवी पिता देवो महेश्वरः |
बान्धवाः शिवभक्ताश्च स्वदेशो भुवनत्रयम् ||12||

Maataa Cha Paarvatii Devii Pitaa Devo Maheshvarah |
Baandhavaah Shiva-Bhaktaash-Cha Svadesho Bhuvana-Trayam ||

My mother is Devi Parvati (Anna Poorna) and my father is
Deva Maheshwara (Shiva).

My friends are the devotees of Shiva, from my country and
all the three worlds.

(FROM *ANNA POORNA STOTRAM* COMPOSED BY
SHRI ADI SHANKARACHARYA)

INTRODUCTION

Food as Friend or Foe?

An Ayurvedic Perspective

My dear readers,

When I was growing up in Jamshedpur, India, we lived a life based on Ayurveda, an ancient system for understanding disease and health that considers food that is grown, cooked, and eaten with reverence as both nutrition and medicine. My parents explained the meaning and purpose of our household rituals and traditions in such a way that we children, six of us, could embrace and carry them forward into our own future. One of my most vivid recollections from my years at my childhood home is the set of rituals my family followed around food, which I now try to emulate. Our parents taught us to talk to the plants that grew year-round in abundance in our front and back kitchen gardens as well as on our rooftop and ask for the plants' forgiveness before cutting, plucking, pruning, or necessarily uprooting them. We were trained to thank the plants for providing us with fruits, vegetables, and flowers and to take only as much as we needed at any given time; thus harvesting was a daily process.

Dhanvantari, the physician to the gods, gave instructions to the rishis and wise sages of ancient India on how to provide a well-balanced and complete medical system for taking care of humans. These details were written down in Sanskrit by the physician Charaka in his Charaka

Samhita treatise and are taught in Ayurvedic medical schools in India. Ayurvedic knowledge for taking care of health has also permeated the culture and has been passed down in familial traditions, and the daily life routines and food habits of many Indians are based on the concepts that have been laid out in Charaka's treatise.

Before we started cooking, my mother would bathe while chanting about the river Ganga. She'd then clean the stove, pots and pans, and kitchen thoroughly and decorate the stovetop and the floor around it with a simple *kolam,* a floral or geometric design made with rice flour. She'd say a prayer to Ganesh, asking him to help the cooking to progress without obstacles, and another to Agni asking him to infuse the food with vital warmth, life, and energy. Because the food would be offered first to God, she never sampled tidbits to ascertain taste, yet she seasoned the food to perfection.

When the food was ready, Mother would carry all the finished dishes to the prayer room and, after lighting the prayer lamp, our parents would chant a prayer to the goddess Annapurna and meditate for a few moments. Then Mother would take out portions for our two cows and their calves, for the birds who visited our garden, and for any person who might come by asking for food. Prior to mealtime, my eldest sister Meenakshi would ensure that all six of us children had taken baths, combed our hair, brushed our teeth, put on fresh, clean clothes, and had a *tilak* (third-eye dot) and *vibhuti* (holy ash) on our foreheads.

After prayers, we would sit on the floor in a semicircle around Mother. Anyone who came by at mealtime was offered food and sent home afterward with a pack of goodies. Picking, criticizing, choosing, or rudely demanding food was not allowed. Our parents explained to us that the food on our plate was made possible by all the plants in our garden working around the clock to produce it, that Mother had cooked the food with devotion because she loved us, that the food had acquired its specific taste and texture because of the grace of Agni, and, finally, that the relationship between food, hunger, and the body remained healthy and normal because of the extreme grace of Ma Annapurna, the universal mother who nurtures all of creation. Thus, they explained, all food is a priceless gift of love from nature and Mother and a symbol of the infinite grace of gods and goddesses. It is Prasad, food offered to God, and it would be a sin to humiliate, neglect, waste, or disrespect food or to express greed, lust, or aggressiveness when eating. It would also be a sin not to share food with other human beings, animals, and birds.

My mother was also a great storyteller, and most of her mealtime stories revolved around concepts like thankfulness, expressing gratitude toward nature and the gods whose grace keeps us in good, physical, mental, and emotional health, and partaking of and enjoying food and benefitting from its life-nurturing qualities. We also saw our parents fast on all religious occasions and for several days every month and donate their share of food to needy people.

My pursuit of academic milestones like master's and doctorate degrees in clinical microbiology took me away from my home in my late teens, and I spent twelve years at two universities, living in dormitories where huge industrial-sized kitchens manufactured food for up to two thousand students at a time. All requirements for a wholesome and pure vegetarian menu were treated with utter disregard. Even in India, the ancient land of pure vegetarianism, the food service believed that providing a vegetarian dish meant removing pieces of meat and serving the leftover potatoes from the same dish.

Being a strict vegetarian, I lived on chapatti (unleavened flatbread) and fruit jams during this time. Nevertheless, every time I sat at the dining table with hundreds of other hungry, angry, complaining, disinterested, hurried, loud, and abusive youngsters, I tried to shut out the noise and visualize the sacred atmosphere around food preparation at our home. I would recall my mother's face that always expressed devotion and love, and then whatever good was in front of me took on special meaning. It became Prasad. My attitude was soon noted by the cooks and servers, and they became quite committed to taking personal care of my vegetarian needs.

When I married a United States–based book publisher and moved to Vermont to begin a family with him, I saw for the first time elaborate nutritional labels printed on the packaging of both raw and prepared food. I saw many people counting calories and fearing some food ingredients as if they were poisons as lethal as cyanide. They appeared to be looking at food with trepidation, suspicion, and fear, as if it were their enemy and would destroy them if they consumed it. They fasted with missionary zeal, but their focus was just on losing weight and flattening abdominal flab. I also read about the various illnesses people got and about how corrective nutritional measures could improve the long-term outcome of these various illnesses regardless of the highly stressed, TV-addicted, and intoxicated state of the population.

Since my childhood in the 1960s, science has reached great milestones by discovering more and more information about food, including its farming, harvesting, storage, transportation, and biochemical nature. Scientists can predict how many calories and how many grams of any particular nutrient consumed might result in greater longevity or a certain amount of muscle mass or bone density and perhaps even predict the perfect diet that would result in that elusive goal: immortality.

But this wealth of information on every material aspect of food seems to have stripped off the reverential, devotional, prayerful, and thankful attitude toward food and ignores the manner in which it is prepared and eaten. It seems that food is seen as a commodity to be consumed daily, and it is often thought to be more of a curse than a blessing. Seeing my parents remain youthful and vigorous into their eighties and nineties and recalling my childhood years at home, it is apparent to me that food's effect on one's body, mind, and soul is connected to one's individual attitude toward growing, harvesting, cooking, sharing, and eating that food.

We are and we become what we eat. This is a well-known Ayurvedic concept that I learned at home from my parents. Ayurveda recognizes that food sustains life by nourishing all five of the known interconnected *koshas,* or sheaths, in the body, which include the *annamaya kosha* (physical body), the *pranamaya kosha* (vital life force), the *manomaya kosha* (mind), the *vijnanamaya kosha* (intellect), and the *anandamaya kosha* (the inner blissful self).[1]

These koshas are like layers in the body, and the *annamaya kosha* is the outermost, gross, material, physical body that is created, maintained, and destroyed by food. If food is taken as a medicine, wisely, judiciously, mindfully, and with an attitude of "eat to live," it can create and maintain a healthy body. However, if food is taken with greed, lust, and a self-indulgent "live to eat" attitude without awareness, knowledge, and refinement, then it destroys the body instead of nurturing and maintaining it.

The *annamaya kosha* is the vessel that carries the other four koshas, and all five koshas are interrelated and affect each other. If one *kosha* is out of balance, it affects the balance and well-being of the other four koshas. For instance, if the *annamaya kosha* is made sick with faulty food, it negatively affects the mind, emotions, feelings, and intellect and also throws a dark veil over the *anandamaya kosha* that is supposed be a source of bliss and light in our lives. Since food can impact our entire being, we truly are, in fact, what we eat, and if we have the desire to become healthier and more energetic, we can do so by changing our interaction with food and by becoming more mindful of what we ingest.

From my childhood background in Ayurveda, I know that the prevention and management of many maladies as well as a cure for some diseases can be accomplished by altering a person's interaction with food and changing what, why, where, when, and how they eat—and sometimes with whom they eat. The latest research in food and nutrition and the insights gained from it suggests that diseases can be prevented and even cured by modification of our eating pattern and the quality of our food.[2] "Food is medicine" is a well-known proverb.

An example from my childhood comes to mind. During Deepavali, the festival of light that is celebrated all over India, we indulged for days at a stretch in very rich, sweet, fried, and to-die-for-delicious festival foods. This festive, overindulgent eating occasionally led to loose stools and vomiting. I recall my mother quoting from the Charaka Samhita, *Langhanam parama aushadham,* which means "Reduction is the ultimate medicine." She explained that overindulgence in rich food causes digestive upset, and that the cure for this malady is simply to reduce the intake of this food.

In her sweet and musical voice, Mother also reminded us of a saying in Tamil:

ஒரு வேளை சாப்பிடுபவன் யோகி
இரண்டு வேளை சாப்பிடுபவன் போகி
மூன்று வேளை சாப்பிடுபவன் ரோகி.

In English this simply means, "One who eats once a day is a yogi, one who eats twice a day is a *bhogi* (a person who likes to enjoy), and one who eats three times a day is *rogi* (a sick individual)."

Never one to worry or suffer from lack of ideas, Mother made us fast for a day after the festival and gave us plenty of warm water to drink. Thereafter, we were offered a small amount of only one type of fruit for breakfast, lunch, and dinner. If we were oversaturated with the sweet taste of the festival foods and declined to eat fruits, then she withheld them and instead made us *kanji* by slow roasting unpolished brown rice containing germ and bran, grinding it into a coarse powder, and then cooking it with sufficient water to give it a soupy texture. For the next two to three days, she served us kanji for all three meals.

Mother's back-to-basics Ayurvedic intervention was very simple and consisted of the following three steps:

1. Withholding or eliminating the problematic food
2. Fasting on water only to flush and cleanse the digestive system

3. Simplifying food intake to one extremely simple, light, and easy-to-digest food

With these three steps, we were able to give the digestive system the much-needed rest from the heavy-duty festival foods and were soon over our upset stomach without any medicine and without having to run to a doctor. Fasting to remove the obstacle to recovery—in this case, rich festival food—allowed the digestive system to automatically correct itself and become healthy again.

This childhood experience of seeing the Ayurvedic principle work like a charm, along with a scientific understanding of industrial foods and modern eating habits and what they do to our health, helped me to see the impact of these practices on our psychosomatic well-being and inspired me to explore the Ayurvedic concept of fasting, isolating foods, and then sensibly combining foods that would work in a modern-day home environment.

Ayurveda is holistic in the sense that it honors and acknowledges the fact that our health as well as our disease states are intrinsically connected to our thoughts, emotions, environment, living conditions, exercise level, and food intake. At the time Ayurveda was developed as a system of medicine thousands of years ago, human beings were still hunting and gathering or conducting small-scale subsistence farming for their basic food needs. Because they depended completely on nature for food, shelter, and medicine, people knew that nature and her rhythms and seasons must be honored.

But times have changed, and people's connection to nature has changed too. We now live in an industrialized world where quantity and profit-driven commerce are valued much more than quality and a benevolent worldview. We have abandoned the peaceful, earth-honoring lifestyle of our ancestors that caused the least amount of harm to the environment and are now paying the price by way of a general decline in our overall health and well-being.

Needless to say, my personal familial background with Ayurveda has helped me see food—its cultivation, preparation, and consumption—from a completely different perspective than the one I hear about from the clients I meet in my Homeopathy practice and what I observe in the modern industrial, commercial methods of cultivating, handling, cooking, and eating food.

Since 2008, I have been engaged in a family practice of Homeopathy. I see many clients with a variety of illnesses. After all, a family practice is an open door for any and all complaints experienced by people. As part of my inquiry into the wellness of my clients, I routinely ask them about their food intake. Finding out about what people eat, how they view their relationship to food, and how they experience food cravings and aversions is part of a general inquiry into the totality of the individual. Some of the food issues people bring to my attention include not being hungry or thirsty, being hungry or thirsty all the time, struggling to lose weight, or losing too much weight too quickly. They eat too much sugar or lick salt off the spoon. They crave chocolate, ice cream, or bread and can easily eat a full bar of chocolate, a pint of ice cream, or a loaf of bread in one sitting. They are into drinking ten or more bottles of soft drinks a day, or they refuse to eat any vegetable that is not white and creamy (i.e., they only eat mashed potatoes).

By inquiring about the client's food habits, it oftentimes becomes as apparent as daylight that at least a part of their wellness concern is connected with faulty food intake. Faulty food and overconsumption of faulty food is helping them to maintain an environment in their body that makes it possible for them to experience varying degrees of sickness.[3] As Thiruvalluvar, a well-known poet-saint from south India, said a few millennia ago, "The pleasures of health abide in the man who eats moderately. The pains of disease dwell with him who eats excessively." Intake of faulty food causes a marked reduction in vitality and bad food habits become an obstacle on the path of recovery and total wellness.

In other words, the uninterrupted overconsumption of bad and lifeless food three times every day with no significant physical activity can cause a myriad of health problems. Lots of faulty and undesirable foods—desserts, ice cream, pastries, baked goods, junk food, and processed foods, snacks, and soft drinks—that are included in many meals can bring in anywhere from 2,500 to 3,000 calories and can be quite unfit for human consumption as we will see in the upcoming chapters. And when these excess calories are not spent in vigorous physical activities, then people begin to see degenerative changes in their body, mind, and spirit—they become prime candidates for the illnesses of the modern times and a vast majority seek recourse for their problems from the medical-pharmaceutical industry instead of taking responsibility for their own health.

Homeopathy in India

In my upbringing my parents used Homeopathy as well as Ayurveda for taking care of their six children. Though Ayurveda has been in use in my country for thousands of years, Homeopathy was introduced in India only during early nineteenth century. Since then, Homeopathy has flourished in India and there are over 195 medical colleges that provide undergraduate education in Homeopathy and 43 that provide postgraduate education, adding over twelve thousand new graduates annually to the pool of practitioners. Over 62 percent of the population in India uses homeopathy exclusively for all its health needs. And the Indian Homeopathic practitioners encounter and treat almost any disease known to humankind.

*For more on how Homeopathy is used to treat disease in India and elsewhere visit the Hpathy website.

Take for example hypertension, cancer, heart disease, and diabetes. The medical community is recognizing now that a highly stressful sedentary life coupled with a diet full of saturated fats and excess salt, red meat, and refined carbohydrates creates an environment in the body that is suitable for the development and maintenance of these diseases.

But all the medicines in the world, taken most diligently, do nothing more than keep symptoms suppressed and expose us to a multitude of side effects, some of them more horrible than the disease itself. They do not cure the problem from the inside out or remove the root cause. This is why people remain on medications for rest of their lives.

Now, I have nothing against doctors! These brilliant people have devoted decades of their lives to studying medical science and are doing their best to help sick people. They can say, "Take this prescription medication and your cholesterol will come down, your blood pressure will be controlled, your sugar will stabilize, your heart valve will work, and you will get longer, harder, better erections," and generally, people will take their advice as word from a higher, more educated, well-meaning, and all-knowing authority. They want to get over their sickness and get on with their lives as quickly as possible, and they hope that if they do exactly what the doctor says and take all the prescribed medications, then their problems will go away. But the best pill prescribed by the very best and brightest doctor is not going to do for you what you must do for yourself.

Understanding the maintaining cause or the obstacle to recovery and removing it requires a sustained discipline on the part of the patient as well as the practitioner. The patient has to *do* something— besides swallowing pills, hopefully—and take charge of their wellness so that they can undo the damage they have inflicted upon themselves from decades of eating bad food and consuming calories over and above their capacity to spend. When the maintaining causes are addressed and removed, the illness either becomes a lot more manageable or goes away completely.

In their Global Burden of Disease study that spanned 195 countries and lasted from 1990 till 2017, researchers from the University of Washington discovered that unhealthy diets cause more deaths than smoking and high blood pressure.[4] They also found that although the consumption of red meat, excess salt, sugary beverages, and other bad foods play a role in the death toll, the majority of deaths are due to people not eating enough of the foods that are good for them—fruits, vegetables, nuts, seeds, and whole grains, for example. By tracking the intake of fifteen different dietary elements, the researchers found that poor diets accounted for 10.9 million deaths worldwide. This is a fifth of the total preventable fatalities. In comparison, tobacco consumption is linked to 8 million deaths and high blood pressure accounts for 10.4 million deaths.

The lead researcher of this study, Ashkan Afshin, has urged the health authorities to focus on promoting healthy eating comprising fruits, vegetables, nuts, seeds, and whole grains and not to stress dropping sugars, fats, and salt. He bases his argument on the logic that when people begin to eat the right kind of food that is good for them, they will drop eating the food that is bad for them. "Generally, in real life people do substitution," he says. "When they increase the consumption of something, they decrease the consumption of other things."[5]

Ayurveda can help anyone to heal the present-day sufferings related to the destruction of humanity's relationship to food and the manner in which it is grown, handled, cooked, and eaten. And you don't have to be particularly spiritual, religious, or holy to reap the benefits of Ayurvedic techniques; they can be used by anyone who needs help, irrespective of their cultural, religious, or spiritual belief systems.

Before you read on about these principles, I want to tell you that Ayurveda has a very vast tool kit at its disposal. It has a system of surgery and a pharmacopoeia that address advanced disease states, and it also has a very strong specialty that deals with preventive measures. The ancient rishis who were scholars and practitioners of Ayurveda knew that an ounce of prevention is worth a pound of cure. To help with the prevention of maladies related to food, Ayurveda recommends a few very simple techniques that anyone can follow in the comfort of their own home and without great expense or any special professional training or intervention. The three simple steps in the time-tested Ayurvedic technique are as follows:

1. Fasting on water only or water and herb teas only to help flush out old remnants, impacted fecal matter, and germs that are harmful and also to rebalance the bacteria in our gut
2. Isolating food by eating only one type of food at a time to simplify digestion and allow the body to fully absorb all the nutrients in a particular food (also known as a mono-diet)
3. Mixing foods from various food groups in a sensible way

Growing up in a household that was based on Ayurveda, I saw first-hand the practicality, utility, simplicity, and intelligence of these three fundamental Ayurvedic principles and how they assist us in regaining vitality. This experience, coupled with the outcome of my inquiry into my client's wellness status and their relationship to food, has motivated me to write this book and place it in your hands.

In the upcoming pages, I will give you a brief history of our hunter-gatherer ancestors and their relationship to seasonal and local foods and tell you about the realities of modern-day food and the problems that are unleashed from *viruddha ahara,* the faulty mixing/combination and intake of food. This information will help you make smart choices about what foods you want to eat. I will also tell you in a step-by-step manner about how to apply the three simple Ayurvedic techniques for taking responsibility for your wellness, because as you may know, self-help is the best help.

To enable you to succeed in your effort, I will explain the physiology of digestion for various food groups like carbohydrates, proteins, and fats so that you can understand the logic behind the Ayurvedic concept of viruddha ahara and why certain types of foods can be a problem when they are mixed/combined. I will also share with you how to shop for fruits, vegetables, and meats from the grocery store, health food store, or your local farmers market, because this is an important piece of the puzzle. You will see how you can completely revise and restructure your pantry, engage in a process of external and internal cleansing, and learn the Ayurvedic technique of eating with all five fingers so that you can satisfy all five of your sensory organs in the process of eating.

All this information will completely equip you to use the three simple Ayurvedic techniques mentioned above in your own day-to-day life and reap the benefits in terms of enhanced and improved wellness. An outstanding feature of these techniques is that while you are busy and fully, diligently, and consciously engaged in healing and rebooting yourself from the inside out, you are not suffering the hunger pangs, exhaustion, deprivation, or cravings that are usually associated with any change in the way we eat or the usual "diet" plans. Instead, you have lightness in the body and a satisfying feeling that finally you are doing something positive, sustainable, and logical to help yourself.

Before I sign off on this message to you, I must emphasize that the Ayurvedic reset diet will keep you supplied with enough abundant energy for your regular day-to-day life and more. So the question is, what do you do with all this energy? Is simply eating the right food at the right time and in right quantity sufficient to keep you healthy? My personal experience is that the energy has to be channeled in a positive direction, and physical exercise and a routine of regular body movement are essential for obtaining the greatest benefit from the Ayurvedic reset diet. Adding an exercise regimen to your day-to-day life will increase the oxygenation and flexibility of the muscles and joints, strengthen the musculoskeletal structures, enhance the blood circulation and waste elimination systems, positively impact moods and emotions, and provide an overall sense of well-being.

It is my earnest hope that this book will give you a fresh perspective on food and that, going forward, you will begin to see food as a friend that helps and supports your efforts to get better and stay better, and not a foe that threatens you and sucks out your vital energy.

HAPPY READING,

VATSALA SPERLING, MS, PH.D., PDHOM, CCH, RSHOM

1

A Season for Everything
The Way Our Ancestors Ate

Bhairav was my father's dear friend and a frequent guest at my childhood home in Jamshedpur, India, during the 1960s. To my eyes, he looked rather different. Bhairav spoke a different language and lived in the forest on the Dalma mountain range just outside the perimeters of the city. That is where all his ancestors, going back a few thousand years, had lived as one with nature.

He had never gone to a formal school, but from living in the forest like his ancestors, he had learned to use a pair of dried twigs to predict the future and had gained an encyclopedic knowledge of how to use various plants and animals as food as well as medicine. His ancestral heritage had taught him to pick medicinal herbs from the forest and use them for healing sick people. He would go on solitary walkabouts in the forest to find answers to questions that our neighbors asked him about their health, wealth, or any particular problems that they might be facing. Our neighborhood considered him a shaman.

My father explained to me that Bhairav was an Adivasi (*adi* = beginning, *vasi* = dweller, or original inhabitant). My father also told me that though India is well known for its very complex and multilayered caste system, the existence of her original inhabitants, the Adivasis, is not generally known. Adivasis were found in almost every state and linguistic region in India, and they were respected and recognized as distinct indigenous tribes by the Hindus of both Dravidian and Aryan origin. In fact, the most famous and enduring epic from India, Ramayana, was written by Sage Valmiki, an Adivasi tribesman-turned-poet. In this epic, when the chief characters—Ram, the prince of Ayodhya; his wife, princess Sita; and his brother Lakshman—were traversing the dense, impenetrable forests of India during the fourteen years of their exile, they met Shabari, an ardent devotee of Ram. Shabari was an elderly Adivasi tribal woman who lived in the forest. She wanted Ram to have the best and sweetest of the berries, so she tasted them first. If they were good and sweet, she would offer them to Ram to eat; if not, she would discard them. Prince Ram, with humility, love, and respect for his devotee, ate the berries that Shabari had bitten into . . . so the story goes.

Just like Shabari, the Adivasi tribes enjoyed complete autonomy; they could use the land and undisturbed primary forests for hunting and gathering and subsistence farming (in recent times), and they were free to maintain their language, social and cultural practices, dances, music, crafts, tool- and pottery-making, and art for making beautiful, clean shelters using mud, dried leaves, logs, and colors available from the earth, plants, or insects. They were known for living in tune with nature, and their spiritual beliefs like animism and Saranaism also mirrored their close relationship with nature. Animism ascribes spiritual powers and potencies to nonhuman components of nature like plants, animals, and minerals. Saranaism is the concept of considering woodlands and forests as holy. With such profoundly naturalistic belief systems, the Adivasi tribes lived in complete harmony with nature, her rhythms and cycles, just as prescribed in Ayurveda, the medical science that originated in India many thousands of years ago.

From 1700 to the mid-1800s the British rulers of India went on a rampage, taking away the land and forests of these autonomous Adivasis and redistributing it among caste Hindus and other Anglophiles for the purpose of consolidating *zamindari*—a feudal system of landholding practiced among high-caste Hindus. These swaths of land were rapidly deforested and put to use in city building, animal husbandry, agriculture, and transportation (railway lines). Missionaries went deep into the woods and converted huge numbers of Adivasis to Christianity.

A way of life that Bhairav and his ancestors had followed for several thousands of years, where man could blend and peacefully coexist and flow with the rhythm and seasons of nature (just as all other animals and plants do) while being completely dependent on nature for food, shelter, and medicine, was eaten away, and their language and culture began to die. Presently, India still has a segment of the population that identifies itself as Adivasi, but their original way of life is gone. However, in Bhairav, I had met at least one pure and ancient Adivasi, and I had seen how he kept the practice of herbal medicine and Ayurveda alive because of his traditional and intimate knowledge of seasons, plants, animals, forests, and minerals and the spiritual energies contained in them.

My parents also told me that thousands of years ago, hunting in the forests was a common practice among Brahmins too. Although the majority of Brahmins in India today are vegetarians, they were known to have consumed meat during their nomadic hunter-gatherer days in the ancient past. This collective cultural memory is enacted during the annual day of remembrance of the dead, *Shraaddh,* when vegetarian dishes representing meat are prepared and offered to the departed ancestors. These foods, served on banana leaves, were not cooked or eaten at any other time of the year or at any other celebration. This memory of hunter-gatherer ancestors was also sung in the Sama Veda and Rig Veda hymns by the Brahmin priests who came to perform the ancestor remembrance ceremony in my home every year.[6] It is mentioned in our scriptures that Sage Agastya had to eliminate demon brothers Vatapi and Ilvala because they used deceit and magic to fool Brahmins into eating meat. Their purpose was to kill the Brahmins.

इह एकदा किल क्रूरो वातापिः अपि च इल्वलः |

भ्रातरौ सहितौ आस्ताम् ब्राह्मणघ्नौ महा असुरौ || ४-११-५५

Once upon a time, verily cruel demon brothers Vatapi and Ilvala were here together, and these dreadful demons, they say, used to be Brahmin killers.

भ्रातरम् संस्कृतम् कृत्वा ततः तम् मेष रूपिणम् |

तान् द्विजान् भोजयामास श्राद्ध दृष्टेन कर्मणा || ४-११-५७

Then Ilvala used to make his brother Vatapi into a ram, perfect that ram's meat into deliciously cooked food, and feed Brahmins according to obsequial rites and deeds.

ततो भुक्तवताम् तेषाम् विप्राणाम् इल्वलो अब्रवीत् |

वातापे निष्क्रमस्व इति स्वरेण महता वदन् || ४-११-५८

When those Brahmins are surfeited with that ram's meat, then Ilvala used to shout loudly, "Oh, Vatapi, you may come out."

ततो भ्रातुर् वचः श्रुत्वा वातापिः मेषवत् नदन् |

भित्त्वा भित्त्वा शरीराणि ब्राह्मणानाम् विनिष्पतत् || ४-११-५९

Then on listening his brother's words Vatapi used to lunge out bleating like a ram, tearing and rending the bodies of those Brahmins.

The collective memory of my ancestors as hunter-gatherers has remained in my mind, and it has been reinforced by the traditions, culture, and religious and ritualistic celebrations around the annual remembrance day for the ancestors, which our family observed diligently.

Mother also told me that according to the Hindu yuga (age) system of understanding the human time line, we are in the Kali Yuga. The very first yuga, Satya Yuga, consisted of 1,728,000 human years. The second, Treta Yuga, had 1,296,000 human years. The third, Dvapara Yuga, had 864,000 human years, and the fourth and final, Kali Yuga, has 432,000 human years. So 1,296,000 + 864,000 = 2,160,000 years ago, in the Satya Yuga, my Hindu ancestors were hunter-gatherers for 1,728,000 years. Agrarian communities were established at the end of the Satya Yuga and beginning of the Treta Yuga. As agrarian settlements were formed, the forests and the flora and fauna living within them began to dwindle. Soon, communities could no longer support themselves with just hunting and gathering, so they gave up the nomadic lifestyle of their hunter-gatherer ancestors, focused completely on raising crops, and became vegetarians by choice.

In fact, cultures on every continent around the world have a collective memory of a time when their ancestors were hunter-gatherers and lived in the forest as a part of nature itself. The Aborigines of Australia, for example, were known to have lived a bucolic, hunter-gatherer lifestyle as recently as the early to mid-1800s, until they were subjugated by the growing number of British convicts and forced to relinquish their way of life.

Before colonization, the Aborigines were able to live according to their own traditions for over 150,000 years, and the earth provided for all their needs. In their worldview, the earth, with all her power, riches, and beauty, was created during Dreamtime, according to the wisdom and power of their ancestors. They lived in it lightly, in complete harmony with the seasons and cycles of nature. Their culture was essentially nomadic; they did not build permanent dwellings and structures, mine, raise crops in fixed-plot agriculture, or weave clothing. However, they had an intimate knowledge of their land, its topography, and its power to provide flora and fauna for their survival and for their health. The hunter-gatherer lifestyle of the Aborigines was completely dependent on the seasons, which affected the availability of their food. They lived as an integral part of nature and did not think themselves any different from the plants and the animals in their environment. All the natural resources belonged to nature. No one owned land, cash, or any other personal property.

The Aborigines did not read and write any language known to Westerners, but they had their own oral tradition and symbols that allowed them to communicate with the members of their tribe about natural resources, and they passed down this information to the younger members of their tribe by way of art, stories, music, and dance. From one generation to the next, they learned the secrets of the land on which they lived. Watering holes, root vegetables and edible flowers, orchards of delicious fruits, and herds of animals were all described in these songs and stories. Children learned to hunt and gather, not by attending any school but by watching the tribal elders in action and by hearing the songs and stories from them about the availability of food directly from nature.

These hunter-gatherer tribes so completely trusted nature to provide for all their needs that they never felt the necessity to hunt and gather even an ounce more than what they could eat in one meal. They did not overeat, hoard, store, process, ferment, preserve, or freeze their foods. They took only what they absolutely needed for survival, fully trusting that nature would provide their next meal. They walked about and foraged in the forest, gathering anything edible that was in season, including nuts, edible flowers, fruits, and vegetables. When an animal species was in abundance, they hunted these animals and ate just meat. Any one type of food that was abundant and in season constituted their main meal and occasionally going without a meal (fasting) was quite okay with them. As seasons changed, different types of animals and plant-based foods became predominant and that is what they ate. They hunted animals, birds, and fish with their simple, wooden, handmade tools. Their unspoiled, natural, and productive land was so fertile, lively, and diverse that it provided for all their needs in the present moment, so they did not have to hoard food for the future.

The Aborigines actually spent very little time hunting and gathering. Once they had eaten, they spent the rest of their day conducting elaborate ceremonies to mark seasons, respect their ancestors, and honor rites of passage; telling stories; dancing; singing; relaxing; and creating abstract art about their ancestral history and the power of their land. They spent their time in quiet contemplation as well as playful interaction with their clan members. They also created rock paintings in their holy sites describing the stories of creation and dreaming that they had learned from their elders.

This natural, peaceful lifestyle respected the earth and nature, and in their 150,000 years of existence, the Aborigines did not deplete, decimate, or destroy their land.[7] This Aboriginal hunter-gatherer lifestyle is quite similar to that of the Adivasi, and both of these old cultures have an innate understanding of the Ayurvedic principles of health and well-being. In fact, Ayurveda was their way of life.

While the ancient Adivasi and Aboriginal tribes were living an idyllic life in the unspoiled forests, totally in tune with nature and her rhythm, farming and animal husbandry practices were beginning in the Indus Valley, about 1,728,000 years ago, according to the Vedic time line. People were beginning to settle down in one place. Cultivating land and raising domesticated animals that could be used for agriculture and meat production required that the farmers take ownership of land, remain in one place, and tend to their land and livestock. During these times, people hunted for some of their foods and also did subsistence farming. They tilled small pieces of land, planted crops, vegetables, and fruits native to the region, and raised animals for meat and labor in their own backyard. Essentially their piece of land provided for the farmer and his family everything that they needed. Although this small-scale hunting, farming, and animal husbandry was contrary to the hunter-gatherer lifestyle, it was still in tune with nature's rhythms.

The farmers had to respect the laws of nature. They could not grow apples in summer and squash in winter. Nature, land, and the resources that they had were used but not exploited. But the population grew, and this lifestyle of hunting and subsistence farming and animal husbandry could not be sustained. To feed the masses, hunting and gathering practices were discontinued and settled, fixed-plot agriculture and large-scale animal husbandry became the norm. In the present era, this progression is seen firsthand in the South American Shuar tribe in the Amazon jungle, where the reduction of natural habitat has eliminated the hunting-gathering practices, and the subsistence farmer is now a professional farmer growing one type of crop.

Western colonization disrupted the harmonious existence of the Adivasi and Aboriginal hunter-gatherers. Aborigines were considered uncivilized and anywhere from ninety thousand to two million of them were killed as Australia was taken over by the British. Over five hundred different languages spoken by the Aborigines were wiped out too. The Europeans brought with them cattle and sheep grazing, agriculture, manufacturing, road and city building, metallurgy, architecture, written language, trade, and commerce as well as arrogance, new diseases, and a juvenile materialistic science that gave them license to desecrate anything that did not fit into their belief system. Globally, on every continent where European civilization arrived, the following events happened:

- Dehumanization, enslavement, displacement, and mass murder of native people
- Decimation of native culture, language, songs, dances, art, stories, traditions, and the relationship of native people to their land
- Destruction of natural flora and fauna
- Exploitation of natural resources and a vicious pattern of constantly taking more than necessary from the earth and not giving it anything in return
- Deforestation to claim land as personal property for fixed plot agriculture, mining, and city building

Similar events of colonization and decimation of ancient hunter-gatherer cultures have been reported in North, Central, and South America, Africa, and parts of Asia.[8] The invaders thought of the natives as brutish and uncivilized barbarians and made sure they would perish from starvation, isolation, disease, and destruction of their natural resources and way of life. The invaders were quite successful in their mission. The ancient way of life that honored and integrated itself with nature has pretty much been wiped out and the "native" people are becoming "civilized," "Westernized," and "modern."

The most outstanding element of the Aboriginal and the ancient tribal Adivasi way of life is that they ate according to the season, because indeed there is a season for everything. They ate what grew on their land. Consuming locally growing, fresh seasonal food was a way of life, and no one had to struggle to do so. Their bodies received wholesome nutrition from live, local, and seasonal foods. They did not import or hoard food. If a particular fruit was in season, they would feast on it and enjoy this particular bounty of nature as long as it lasted. When the season was over and this fruit was not available anymore, they ate the next food that was available. Because of this practice, the diversity of their diet was controlled by nature, and every meal was natural, fresh, and completely healthy.

Fasting was a regular practice among these ancient people and is what nature intends for us modern people as well, because we are also simply a tiny part of the complex, interconnected web of life. It turns out that this is how wild animals live in nature too. They hunt or forage, eat what they are able to get, and in lean times or after a big eating frenzy, they reduce their food intake. Fasting for extended periods of time is built into their natural rhythm.

European settlers started turning the native tribes into farmers and employed slaves to carry out hard labor in the fields and mines, requiring them to work very long hours. Just to get the maximum amount of work done, they fed the tribal people and slaves three meals a day so that they would have enough energy for hard labor.[9] Now, the need for hard physical labor is gone from most of our lives, but the routine of eating three full meals has remained with us. The easy availability of industrially grown and processed foods, electricity, refrigeration, and long work hours all contribute to continuing the habit of three meals a day.

Compare this to hunter-gatherer eating habits and the less reliable availability of hunted meats and gathered fruits, nuts, root vegetables, and wild grains, which often meant going hungry for long durations when hunting expeditions were unsuccessful or when fluctuations in temperature and rainfall reduced the amount of food that could be gathered. In these "lean years," the people ate one meal a day.

The question that might come to mind here is, how can we possibly go back to the lifestyle of our hunter-gatherer ancestors? We are sons and daughters of the moment. We have a lifelong habit of eating three meals a day and snacking in between. How can we turn away from a habit so deeply ingrained in the collective culture and psyche of our time? No one can ever go back to the past.

This is where Ayurveda can step in to help. The Ayurvedic techniques described in this book will allow you to start your own program now, in this present moment, that will help your body heal. No matter where you are in your life, you can take the following three Ayurvedic principles to heart and practice them:

1. Fast from time to time to reboot your body.[10]
2. Live your life in harmony with nature by eating small amounts of simple foods that grow or can be hunted in season, because indeed there is a season for everything.
3. Combine food sensibly so that your body is better able to draw complete nutrition from the food you eat.

The chapters ahead provide simple, practical tools that will enable you to implement these Ayurvedic techniques into your life.

2

The New Normal

Loss of Seasonality and Quality in Modern Eating

Before we learn how to apply the Ayurvedic techniques, let us first see why we need to even consider them.

In the modern era, advances in industrial technologies enabled curious and adventurous people from every European nation to travel to lands they had never known existed. A process of global colonization began, and international trade routes were established crisscrossing the seas and the skies around the world. These trade routes facilitated large-scale migrations and a dispersal of food crops and introduced nonindigenous animals to new environments. These same trade routes also allowed for human trafficking and the relocation of millions of people from their native lands to new places. For example, about twelve million Africans were brought to the United States between the sixteenth and nineteenth centuries and sold into slavery.

The subjugation and annihilation of ancient tribes and their hunter-gatherer or subsistence-farming lifestyles, cultures, and traditions, along with malicious exploitation and destruction of nature herself, became a trend. Charles Darwin's theory of evolution gave license to the European nations to put themselves on top of the evolutionary chain, and they set the trends for the front line of business, commerce, culture, tradition, fashion, food, and even education. The people of old lands, old cultures, and old traditions were forced to give up their ancient ways, and they had no choice but to imitate and emulate the colonizers or perish while protesting.

MASS PRODUCTION AND TRANSPORTATION OF FOOD

The industrial revolution facilitated the formation of industries, mechanization, and mass production of goods. People began to give up subsistence farming and, en masse, migrated from rural areas to cities to work in manufacturing jobs. During this time and increasingly throughout the subsequent century subsistence farming gave way to industrial farming using machines, and farmers could own and cultivate thousands of acres of land. The spread of electricity, improvement of steam trains and ocean liners, and improvement of automobiles enabled mass movement of edible goods from where they were produced to the cities where people congregated by the millions to earn a living in their industrial manufacturing jobs. The discovery of refrigeration, freezing, and bottling/packaging techniques combined with fast-paced transportation technology ensured that food grown in the rural farmland could reach the city dwellers.

The transportation of food meant that city dwellers no longer needed to grow their own food. Prime real estate and multistory apartment buildings in the cities did not allot any piece of land to city people for farming, so they had to satisfy their need for growing things with container gardening if they were interested at all. While performing their industrial manufacturing jobs for eight to ten hours a day, city dwellers forgot all about the seasons, nature, and the hunter-gatherer/subsistence-farming lifestyle that were an inseparable part of life for their ancestors just a few generations before. They forgot how to grow their own food. They forgot how to slaughter their own animals for food or catch a fish. They even forgot how to raise chickens! They now simply went to the store to purchase food with the wad of cash they had stuffed in their wallet.

YEAR-ROUND AVAILABILITY OF NONSEASONAL FOOD

Industrial farming led to the overproduction and year-round availability of foods that we now experience. New methods of preparation and packaging of ready-to-eat foods have become a boon to supermarkets and city dwellers, and the constant supply of these foods does not depend on the season. One example is rice cultivation in India. Traditionally, rice is planted just before the monsoon rain season. When the monsoon rains arrive in June/July, the newly germinated plants are transplanted into fields of ankle-deep water. When the rainy season is over (October/November) and drier, cooler weather comes in, the rice kernels fill out and mature. Then rice is harvested in December/January. However, revolutionary industrial and scientific developments created rice varieties that grow and mature in just ninety days, and the farmer can get three crops every year instead of just one. Overproduction means that if the harvested rice is preserved and stored well, it can be available year-round and thus rice has become a staple food in the country. The same is true of wheat. It is available year-round because of industrial agriculture, transportation, and storage practices.

The shelf life of staple and ready-to-eat foods is enhanced using methods and systems developed by the food industry. For better shelf life, the staples depend on the heavy use of chemicals that deter pests and prevent mold. Ready-to-eat or packaged foods, on the other hand, have a very long shelf life because during manufacturing, artificial colors and flavors, preservatives, and many chemicals are used to enhance taste and appearance. These foods are drowned in sugar, salt, and hydrogenated fats. From cultivation all the way through the mass manufacturing and display process, the supermarket foods are stripped of natural micronutrients, fibers, enzymes, and vitamins. An industrially grown, processed, and packaged food available in the supermarket has a minimum amount of natural nutrients and simply contains calories from sugars and fats.

The industrial manufacturing process makes it possible to obtain all types of food all year round. Every type of food is available in every supermarket in the country and in every country of the world. This is the true expression of globalization. You can buy mangos in Alaska in the dead of winter. You can buy ice cream in the Sahara, black beans in the Himalayas, and vegetable samosas in the South Pole. The food industry tricks people into believing that they are buying food. In truth, they are spending their hard-earned money on industrially produced goods that are nothing but a compilation of toxic ingredients cooked, packaged, and made to look like food.

A city-based lifestyle also ensures that though people get tired from their repetitive routine jobs and spending time in traffic, crowds, and noise, they do not get sufficient and good quality physical exercise. Their industrial or desk-bound office jobs do not allow them any time in nature or even exposure to sunlight, and this increases their physical and physiological stress levels. In addition, when people eat the same nutritionally dead food year-round, their body quickly learns that there is no other source of nutrition and in order to get all the essential nutrients, it begins to depend on the consumption of greater and greater quantities of the same monotonous food. What is lost in quality is searched for in quantity.

The difference between ancient and modern life can be understood by comparing this eating style to the food habits of our hunter-gatherer ancestors. They lived as part of nature. They hunted and gathered for every meal and took the very minimum of what was available and in season. They ate raw food and did not cook, preserve, ferment, store, hoard, or purchase it. Their food was 100 percent natural and wholesome in the sense that it contained all the nutrients needed for the development, growth, and repair of the body in sufficient quantities.

They did not experience food shortage and hunger as modern city people do who live on store-bought foods that are deficient in nutritional quality.

The modern lifestyle supported by the industrialization of food production is in fact 100 percent opposite to how our ancestors lived. It has nothing to do with season or locality. It is produced and sold for profit, and it is purchased out of fear of not having food available for the next meal. It is preserved using chemicals, shoved into the fridge and freezer, and overcooked, microwaved, baked, fried, refried, heated, and reheated a countless number of times. And people have to eat a huge amount of food to get the minimum amount of nutrition. For example, the simple carbohydrates available in a slice of bread made from refined flour that contains no fiber are digested so quickly that the released sugars are rapidly absorbed in the bloodstream, and very soon after eating such a slice of bread, we want to eat something more, or we want additional slices of the same bread. Our hunger and need for nutrition are not satisfied by a slice of bread made from ultra-refined white flour.

On the other hand, a slice of bread made from unrefined flour has natural fibers that take much longer to digest. As a result, the sugars from digestion of the bread's carbohydrates take much longer to absorb fully in the bloodstream, and we do not feel hungry soon after eating such a slice of bread.

The bottom line of industrial manufacturing of food is *profit for the manufacturer and loss of seasonality and local, natural, wholesome food for the consumer.* It is not a win-win situation.

EATING OUT

A city-based lifestyle also promotes a phenomenon called "eating out." People eat out for various reasons. They get tired after work and have no interest, time, or energy to cook their own food, so they spend their extra cash on restaurant foods. They may also feel too lazy to shop for groceries; carry the bags home; put the food away in their pantry; cut, chop, mince, slice, and clean the various ingredients; and do whatever else is required for food preparation.

There are many restaurants out there, and they serve food in every price range and from every continent on earth, so they provide the appearance of diversity and a feeling of cosmopolitan sophistication. People who know nothing about India or the spices that grow there can enjoy a curry dish and Hyderabadi biryani. And Indians who do not know much about China can enjoy a dish of dim sum, wonton soup, or Kung Pao chicken.

Because restaurants cook and serve food for our taste buds and not for our health, they use refined ingredients, colors, preservatives, salt, sugar, and fat in the maximum amount necessary for great taste. Their foods, to some people at least, look and taste better than home-cooked foods. The ambiance and décor of restaurants are designed to whip up an appetite, and the waiters serve food with good manners and decorum (at least in high-end restaurants). This gives the diners an experience of novelty, class, opulence, and luxury. With a little bit of extra cash on hand, they can get all of these, so why struggle to cook at home and bother with cleaning the dishes afterward?

Here are some survey statistics on the restaurant habits of Americans:[11]

- 20 percent visit a quick-service restaurant once a week
- 20 percent visit a full-service restaurant once a week
- 25 percent regularly dine out in coffee shops
- 11 percent eat out with friends once a week
- 9 percent eat out with family once a week
- 8 percent eat out with a partner once a week
- 10 percent eat out alone once a week

Eating out, then, is a major modern pastime, and it is completely divorced from the concept of seasonality and eating for good health. This phenomenon is based on available cash, a lack of time, interest, energy, and space for cooking wholesome foods at home, and the desire to dress up and sit in a comfortable, stimulating restaurant setting and be served by waiters without having to clean the kitchen or do any dishes afterward.

However, in my childhood in India in the 1960s, restaurants were few and far between. People ate whatever their grandmother, mother, and aunts cooked at home. In my community, eating out was not even considered kosher because profit-driven restaurants paid the least amount of attention to Ayurvedic principles for cooking food. So we did not eat out. All our fruits and vegetables were grown by our family in our own kitchen garden, our staples were sourced from local farmers, and our dairy came from a couple of our own cows. We ate vegetarian food and had no need for eggs, poultry, meat, or seafood. Every food item was sourced from within a hundred miles of where we lived.

The High Price of Eating Out

One popular fast-food restaurant is McDonald's, where many diners order hamburgers in various sizes, including the Big Mac. This meal is available 365 days a year in McDonald's locations all over the world and is so popular that Americans coined the phrase "Big Mac attack," meaning that the desire to eat a Big Mac has taken over their mind—has attacked them—and now they must find the nearest McDonald's so they can eat one.

Here is a list of ingredients in the bun alone:

Enriched flour (bleached wheat flour, malted barley flour, niacin, reduced iron, thiamin, mononitrate, riboflavin, folic acid), water, high fructose corn syrup and/or sugar, yeast, soybean oil and/or canola oil, contains 2% or less of the following: salt, wheat gluten, calcium sulfate, calcium carbonate, ammonium sulfate, ammonium chloride, dough conditioners (may contain one or more of the following: sodium stearoyl lactylate, datem [diacetyl tartaric acid of esters of mono and diglycerides], ascorbic acid, azodicarbonamide, mono- and diglycerides, ethoxylated monoglycerides, monocalcium phosphate, enzymes, guar gum, calcium peroxide), sorbic acid, calcium propionate and/or sodium propionate (preservatives), soy lecithin.[12]

Instead of using all these ingredients, simple buns can be made at home with flour, salt, yeast, and water. The extra chemical ingredients are not needed by your body and can actually be harmful. Take, for example, just a few of the items from the list:

- Ammonium chloride—Used in making fireworks, safety matches, and contact explosives. This chemical is on the New Jersey Department of Health's "Right to Know Hazardous Substance List." It can irritate the skin, nose, throat, and lungs; damage the eyes; and cause asthma and like allergies, and it may affect the kidneys as well.
- Ammonium sulfate—Used most commonly as a fertilizer for alkaline soils. It's also in flame-retardant materials. Ammonium sulfate activates yeast, so it helps to get industrially produced bread to rise. This chemical can irritate the skin, eyes, and respiratory system and is deemed harmful if swallowed.
- Soybean and/or canola oil—Most likely made from genetically modified seeds, which animal studies indicate are harmful to humans indicated in toxic reactions in the digestive tract, liver and other organ damage, reproductive failure, infant mortality, immune reactions, and allergies. In addition, these oils release cancer-causing free radicals under high heat and the refining process they go through involves either very high temperatures or damaging chemicals. Soybean oil has also been linked to metabolic and neurological conditions.
- High fructose corn syrup—Used in almost all processed foods, so it is hard to avoid, but it is very harmful. It is found to cause

inflammation, obesity, diabetes, heart diseases, and cancer.

- Enriched flour—"Enriched" means that all the nutrition was taken out and then some of it was added back in chemical form. Refined flours digest very rapidly so you feel hungry more quickly, and because all fiber is removed, the refined flour, though "enriched," does not move easily through the intestines, which often leaves you constipated.

Many of the rest of the ingredients in the bun are also detrimental to health, and the hamburger, onion, cheese, lettuce, and pickle used for assembling the meal are mass produced using chemical fertilizers, pesticides, herbicides, artificial colors, harmful hormones, and so on. They are transported thousands of miles and come to us unfit for human consumption.

Please note that the list of ingredients does not disclose their places of origin, but we can make an educated guess. Wheat for the bun is quite likely grown in China, and the buns are probably also made in a bun factory in China. Cattle are raised in Brazil. Potatoes are grown in Idaho. Soybean oil and lard come from Vietnam where rain forests have been decimated to make room for growing genetically engineered soybeans and housing pig factories. Sugar is from Brazil, salt from the Netherlands, and water for making Coca-Cola from the ground waters in rural India. America supplies all the chemical fertilizers, genetically engineered seeds, preservatives, pesticides, insecticides, artificial colors, antibiotics, and whatever else is needed in producing, distributing, and marketing this toxic meal to every country in the world. Is this real food? Is it local? Is it seasonal? Which hunter-gatherer or subsistence-farming tribe could have imagined that one day their descendants living and working in the city would be paying to purchase this garbage that is sold as food?

To summarize, the modern phenomenon of a city-based lifestyle relies completely on the highly processed, industrially manufactured food sold in the supermarkets. The food is always the same, irrespective of the season, and it is usually grown thousands of miles away from where it is eaten. The steep price we have paid for this reliance is the loss of fresh, delicious, and nutritious seasonal food and with it, the loss of prana (energy), vitality, and overall good health.

For these reasons alone, the simple Ayurvedic technique of fasting to reboot our body (after years of ingesting faulty food), eating one type of simple food at a time, and then combining compatible foods in a sensible manner becomes a must for our well-being as you will read in chapters 4 through 7. In the next chapter, however, we will take an in-depth look at the food production industry so that you can learn facts to enable you to make better decisions about the food you choose to eat.

3
Industrial Food Production
Technology for Taming and Manipulating Nature

Dear readers,

I just want to alert you to the fact that this chapter does contain some disturbing details of industrial food production. Some of these facts you might know; some might be new to you.

I wish to emphasize here that time, as we understand it, only moves forward. We cannot possibly go back in time and live in the past; we can only live in the present moment. And in this moment, the details of industrial food production are gory indeed. Modern food production includes mechanization, dehumanization, cruelty, exploitation, shortsightedness, greed, and every other negative quality that you can imagine. Presently, these attributes connected with modern food production are here to stay; they cannot be wiped clean, wished away, or made to disappear.

As you read this chapter, please be aware that although time cannot be turned back, you can at least understand what you are putting into your body as food. How your food is grown or slaughtered is an important piece of information that will allow you to make informed choices as you spend your hard-earned money on food.

Although industrial food production is as harmful to the planet as all the known diseases unleashed all at once would be to humankind, the best you can do in the given circumstances is to educate yourself about the origin of your food and steer clear of toxic mass-market food as much as possible. This is something you can do for your health and well-being, since you cannot practically go back in time and live the life of a hunter-gatherer.

Again, always be aware about what you purchase as food and what you put in your mouth as food. It is impossible to completely avoid eating some of the industrially manufactured foods and ingesting all the toxic chemicals they contain, but there are things you can do to help yourself, and practicing the Ayurvedic reset diet is one of them.

Although our ancient ancestors lived a lifestyle that allowed them to blend with nature, becoming one with its seasons and cycles and using the minimum of its nonhuman components for food, shelter, and medicine, modern-day industrial food production, including both plant- and animal-based foods, revolves around the concept of *flood of quantity and drought of quality*. It is based on taming and manipulating nature, and it also creates a harmful environmental footprint that is hard to erase.

GRAINS, LEGUMES, FRUITS, AND VEGETABLES

A small-scale subsistence farmer could grow what his family needed and do so with full respect for the seasons and his land. One area of his plot could have corn and beans, another area could have spinach, onions, cucumbers, and peppers, and the rest of the space could be filled with lemon and papaya trees. Using all the refuse from his land, he could make compost in his backyard. A little pond could help him water his crops and also raise fish and ducks for the family. A few hens could give him all the eggs he and his family needed, and a cow could provide them with milk. In the next season, he could plant a different type of crop. He could also use some of his produce to barter with his neighbor who might be growing different kinds of food crops.

In contrast, a commercial farmer becomes a specialist in one particular crop. He has to grow food for people he has nothing to do with. The more he grows, the more cash he can earn. Subsistence farming is not sustainable for him anymore. Farmers have to learn to create hybrid crops and use farming machinery and industrially produced chemical fertilizers, insecticides, herbicides, and preservatives for long-term storage of their crop in industrial warehouses. A farmer now has to become a professional who specializes in one crop such as potatoes, rice, wheat, sugarcane, and so on. He has forgotten the fact that by cultivating a small patch of land according to the season, he can feed his family. Instead he has become dependent on cash to purchase things he has forgotten how to grow.

Monoculture, a system of planting the same crop year after year on the same land, has successfully depleted the natural nutrients of the soil. For example, a hybrid variety of genetically engineered wheat grown every year on the same piece of land and inundated with chemical fertilizers, herbicides, insecticides, and pesticides provides a greater yield of wheat per hectare of land than a more natural, unmodified wheat, but it is nutritionally dead. It is loaded with toxic chemicals, and it cannot be easily digested by the human body. It looks like wheat, but it has none of the nutrients of wheat anymore. This decimation of nutrients and enhancement of toxicity has happened to most of the commercially grown food crops—grains, legumes, fruits, and vegetables—that are available year-round in the supermarkets.[13]

The following is a list of the harmful effects of modern-day industrial agriculture practices:[14]

- Soil quality becomes depleted due to monoculture. Because toxic chemicals are used excessively to produce a single type of crop, the industrial farmland does not support earthworms and beneficial bacteria.

- Genetically modified crops cross-pollinate with other nonmodified natural crops and create unsustainable gene pools.
- Plants become dependent on herbicides, fungicides, and insecticides for their very survival because they are not allowed to develop natural resistance to the harmful substances of their environment.
- The chemicals used to fend off insects and pests remain in the crop as residue and become part of the human body when they are consumed. They also leach into groundwater reservoirs, rivers, streams, and lakes and reach the oceans as well to impact marine life.
- Pests that are constantly exposed to the *Bacillus thuringiensis* toxin (Bt) that is genetically embedded in crops will become resistant to it, and the efficacy of Bt as a natural pesticide will come to an end.
- Farmers who buy genetically engineered terminator seeds (seeds that produce plants that bear sterile seeds) end up raising crops that do not yield viable seeds for the next season, so farmers have to buy new seeds every year. This practice supports an agricultural monopoly by agribusinesses that create a lot of environmental harm.
- Although 60 percent of all industrial foods in the United States contain genetically engineered products, most consumers will not be able to identify them because the manufacturer is not required to disclose this fact on the label.

ANIMALS AS SOURCES OF FOOD

The exploitation of animals for food production is an even darker story. There was once a time when every farm and many suburban households had a few chickens, ducks, cows, and pigs scavenging in the yard, getting some household scraps and sometimes a handful of grain each day. This method of farming is called extensive, and the number of these farms has decreased as intensive industrialized farming methods have developed, allowing one person to care for large numbers of animals. Animals raised for food are considered a commodity and handled almost as if they are lifeless. Factory farming of animals does not treat them as living beings who can feel any pain, and as a result, they are treated with utmost cruelty.

CHICKENS AND EGGS

It is estimated that over 60 percent of the world's eggs are produced in industrial settings, and more than 300 million chickens work full time in barren battery cages to produce millions of eggs that are eaten as a breakfast staple. Each barren battery cage accommodates at least ten birds, and each bird is allowed the space equivalent to a standard letter-size sheet of paper (8.5 x 11 inches) where it can barely stand. The European Union banned barren battery cages in 2012, but this style is widely practiced in the rest of the world, including the United States.

Several of these batteries are stacked one on top of the other in sheds that house tens of thousands of birds in artificially illuminated and ventilated areas. Caged hens never get to experience natural light or fresh air. They are imprisoned in cages until they are taken to slaughter. Modern commercial hens have been bred to produce large numbers of eggs. A combination of severely restricted bodily movement (i.e., lack of exercise) and a depletion of the hen's store of calcium can result in high occurrences of osteoporosis and fractures. It is impossible to inspect every single bird when they are housed in a large number of tiered cages, so sick and injured birds die unnoticed. Frustrated birds peck at the cage and peck at each other, losing a large amount of their feathers. To prevent feather pecking, chicks often have part of their beaks cut off, and since using an anesthetic agent would add to the cost, they are debeaked without anesthesia. Even today, in the United States, debeaking is done using blades or infrared light.

It goes without saying that these factory hens have never met or said hello to a rooster and never even heard his call. They are given grains, antibiotics, and hormones that keep them perpetually in an egg-producing phase. And against their natural instincts, they can never fly or climb, nor can they brood their eggs or ever have a few chicks of their own to raise and nurture. Their life is all about laying eggs in the most mechanized and cruel conditions, and once they have served their purpose, if they do not get sick and die in the cage, they are sent for slaughter.

Annually, Americans eat over nine billion broiler chickens. The fate of broiler chickens is no different from that of their egg-laying sisters. Broiler chickens also spend their entire lives in crowded sheds with millions of other birds, get sick from overcrowding, and die before their time. They are bred and medicated to grow very large, but their body cannot keep up with such an accelerated growth, and they are prone to heart attacks and organ failure and become crippled under their own weight. At six to seven weeks of age, they are sent out for slaughter.[15]

DAIRY COWS

Cows are intelligent and playful mammals. They love to socialize in their herd and nurture their calves with colostrum and milk. They are placid, patient, peaceful, and nonaggressive animals, and anyone who has raised cows will know that each cow has a unique and distinct personality and is capable of showing a wide range of emotions. But most cows raised for the dairy industry are intensively confined, as if they are in a high security prison. They are not allowed to fulfill their most basic desires, such as mating with a real bull and nursing their calves, even for a single day. They are considered milk-producing machines and are genetically manipulated and pumped full of antibiotics and hormones in order to increase milk production. Their spines get bent out of shape from the weight of their unnaturally large udders. They are given a nonstop supply of artificial food that will increase the protein and fat content of milk. Cows produce milk to nourish their calves—but calves on dairy farms are separated from their mothers when they are just one day old. They are fed milk replacers (including cattle blood) so that their mothers' milk can be sold in the supermarkets. Female cows are artificially inseminated shortly after their first birthdays. After giving birth, they lactate for ten months and are then inseminated again, continuing the cycle, and as a result, they are constantly pregnant and producing milk.

Cows have a natural lifespan of about twenty years and can produce milk for eight or nine years. However, the factory farming techniques make them sick prematurely and at about four or five years of age, they are sent to be slaughtered. In the United States, milk production has increased from 116 billion pounds of milk per year in 1950 to 206 billion pounds in 2014, though the number of dairy cows has come down. Normally, cows would produce just enough milk to meet the needs of their calves, but genetic manipulation—and, in some cases, antibiotics and hormones—is used to cause each cow to produce more than 20,000 pounds of milk each year. Cows are also fed unnatural, high-protein diets—which can include chicken feathers and fish—because their natural diet of grass would not provide the nutrients that they need to produce such massive amounts of milk.[16]

Continuous mechanical lactation leads to painful inflammation of mammary glands, or mastitis. Milk from dairy cows is subjected to somatic cell count (SCC) to determine whether the milk is infected with somatic cells, which include white blood cells, produced for combating infection, and skin cells that are normally shed from the lining of the udder. The SCC of healthy milk is below 100,000 cells per milliliter. The dairy industry is allowed to combine milk from all the cows in a herd in order to arrive at a "bulk tank" SCC, or BTSCC. Milk with a maximum BTSCC of 750,000 cells per milliliter can be sold. A BTSCC of 700,000 or more generally indicates that two-thirds of the cows in the herd are suffering from mastitis. Better living and milking conditions can overcome this problem, but instead the dairy industry is exploring the use of cattle that have been genetically manipulated to be resistant to mastitis.[17]

BEEF CATTLE

Beef cattle are allowed to spend the first six to eight months of their lives grazing, and they get to satisfy some of their natural urges, but they graze within a restricted area and suffer from extreme weather conditions, including heat, cold, and seasonal floods. They can also be attacked by predators. U.S. wildlife agencies have to kill thousands of wild animals each year to protect the cattle. Such elimination of wildlife disrupts the ecosystem and food chain.

After several months of grazing, cattle are moved to confined feedlots where they are meant to gain weight at an incredible speed. Some large animal-feeding locations can house up to a hundred thousand cattle. Over the next six to eight months, they are given high-protein grain-based feed consisting of corn, soy, and miscellaneous by-products, some of which come from animal sources that cattle do not eat naturally. According to the latest FDA guidelines, cattle feed can include nonmammalian protein sources as well as chicken manure. All the ingredients of the cattle's food are treated with various chemicals, which ultimately accumulate in the cattle's tissues. Cattle's stomachs are highly specialized for breaking down grasses. Eating non-grass processed food causes them a lot of digestive complications.

Approximately 90 percent of the industrially farmed U.S. cattle have growth hormones added to their feed. The scientific community is concerned that several of the hormones could potentially cause serious health complications in humans. The European Union has banned the use of growth hormones in domestic beef production, as well as the importation of hormone-treated beef because the consumption of this beef has the potential of creating endocrinal, developmental, immunological, genetic, neurobiological, and carcinogenic effects in humans. However, the U.S. government claims that the hormone residues in beef are harmless to human health.

In addition to growth hormones, industrially farmed cattle are treated with antimicrobials (including antibiotics). The antibiotics are administered for both therapeutic and nontherapeutic purposes. Therapeutic treatments are given in a preventative manner to keep the animal from becoming ill due to the increased presence of bacteria in their unnatural living conditions. Therapeutic antibiotics also help to keep the animals' immune system artificially boosted while they endure an unnatural level of stress throughout their lives. Nontherapeutic treatments act similar to growth-promoting hormones and help to increase weight.

Fourteen- to sixteen-month-old cattle are force-fed to grow and once they have reached the ideal weight of twelve hundred pounds, they are slaughtered. They do not get to live their natural lifespan. During transportation, which can last anywhere from a few hours to a few days, they get motion sickness but are not given food, water, or rest. They vomit and have loose stools from fear as they proceed to the slaughterhouse. At the slaughterhouse, they are stunned into unconsciousness and their throats are cut. Some regain consciousness while being bled out, but they are processed for meat anyway.

More than thirty-four million cattle are slaughtered each year in the United States. Throughout their lives, these gentle animals are treated cruelly with regard to food and housing. They get sick and are mutilated, and their suffering ends only when they die or are killed in the slaughterhouse.[18]

VEAL: MEAT FROM CALVES

Female calves are kept alive for milk or beef production. Male calves are separated from their mothers when they are as young as one day old to be chained in tiny stalls for three to eighteen weeks and raised for veal. They are fed a milk substitute that is designed to make them gain at least two pounds per day, and they are given a low-iron feed so that they become anemic and their flesh stays pale. In addition to becoming sick and lame, these young calves are terrified and desperate for their mothers.[19]

PORK

If you have watched pigs grow or have read about Wilbur, the pig in *Charlotte's Web,* you know that pigs are clean, intelligent, and playful animals that can live into their teens. They are quite protective of their young ones, and they form strong bonds with their caretakers and with other pigs in their group. However, only in the movies do pigs get to run around and play with other pigs. In the United States alone, 115 million pigs are killed for food each year.

Breeding sows are artificially impregnated at seven months of age, and then they spend the rest of their lives in a hormonally induced cycle of pregnancy, birth, and nursing till they are eventually sent to slaughter. Once pregnant, they spend all their time confined in the gestation crates and have to lie on cold, wet, and feces-covered cement floors. After giving birth, they are allowed to nurse their piglets briefly, but they cannot build nests for their piglets as they would otherwise do in nature, and nursing piglets are separated from mothers when they are ten days old.

This intensive confinement produces stress hormones, and sows exhibit stress-induced behaviors such as chewing cage bars, obsessively pressing against water bottles, and displaying learned helplessness, such as remaining passive when poked or when a bucket of water is poured over them. They get sick with mouth sores, skin sores, repeated urinary tract infections, diarrhea, respiratory infections, excessive heat loss, loss of bone density, loss of muscle tone, cardiovascular diseases, foot injuries, joint damage, and lameness.

In this imprisoned, unhappy life, the only thing that they are assured of is a constant supply of grain-based foods for weight gain, hormones for reproduction, antibiotics for various infections, water for drinking and plumping up flesh, and the constant company of their own excreta. Pigs and piglets are subjected to the same cruelty as cattle.[20]

ENVIRONMENTAL IMPACT OF ANIMAL HUSBANDRY

Large dairy farms have an enormously detrimental effect on the environment. In California, America's top milk-producing state, manure from dairy farms has poisoned hundreds of square miles of ground-water, rivers, and streams. Each of the more than one million cows on the state's dairy farms excretes eighteen gallons of manure daily. Overall, factory-farmed animals, including those on dairy farms, produce 1.65 billion tons of manure each year, much of which ends up in waterways and drinking water. The Environmental Protection Agency reports that agricultural runoff is the primary cause of polluted lakes, streams, and rivers. The dairy industry is the primary source of a smog-forming pollutant (33 to 176 metric tons of ammonia gas per day) in California, and a single cow emits more of these smog-forming gases than a car does.

Two-thirds of all agricultural land in the United States is used to raise animals for food or to grow genetically engineered grain to feed them. As massive quantities of manure are dispersed as fertilizer, residues from the growth hormones and antibiotics leech from the manure and end up in local streams and lakes. The chemicals can have a devastating effect on freshwater ecology—especially fish and amphibians. Antibiotic- and hormone-laced feces and urine from millions of factory-raised pigs is dumped into rivers and sewage pits, and this leads to the contamination of ground and surface water as well as air.[21]

Raising animals for food also requires massive amounts of water. Each cow raised by the dairy industry consumes as much as forty gallons of water per day. A single pig needs five gallons of water daily. While growing to market weight, each pig consumes more than 500 pounds of grain, corn, and soybeans.

To constantly fulfill the demands of meat, milk, and agricultural products, the American industrial giants began using the natural resources of South and Central America. As a result, many millions of acres of primary rainforest are lost annually in the Amazon area and other Latin American countries.[22] This primal land has been deforested, and the native species of flora and fauna lost. The land is now used for the industrial production of crops, meat, and milk, so South American countries have not only lost the land, they have incurred all the environmental hazards that come with industrial farming and animal husbandry as well.

IMPACT OF INDUSTRIALLY MANUFACTURED FOOD ON PHYSICAL HEALTH

It is easy to understand that the industrial farming of food crops as well as animals is as far from natural as possible. It is about producing great quantities of low quality and highly polluted foods. In this modern style of food production, technology is used to tame and manipulate nature, and such interference also changes the character of the food: it looks like food, but it fails to nourish us physically and psychologically. The regular supermarkets, driven by a motive for profit and the compulsion to provide food throughout the year, ignore the issues of quality and stock up their shelves with food that is toxic to consumers. These mass-produced industrial foods are not manufactured for ensuring good health, and in fact consuming them for years on end sets a very good stage for food-related illnesses.

Take, for example, the problems associated with drinking milk. The majority of species stop drinking milk after infancy because once they've reached a certain age, they can no longer digest it. Most people begin to produce less lactase, the enzyme that helps with the digestion of milk, when they are as young as two years old, yet they continue to drink cow's milk throughout their childhood and often into adulthood, which can lead to health issues.

According to the American Gastroenterological Association, processed cow's milk and milk powders are the number one cause of food allergies among infants and children. Ultra-pasteurized cow's milk is devoid of the natural bacteria that produce lactase, the enzyme that helps us digest the lactose in milk.[23] Dispersion of milk fat into the milk by the method of homogenization ensures that the fat molecule is broken and can no longer be digested naturally. Instead, it accumulates in the body as extra layers of fat. Also, the removal of milk fat and the making of fat-free, low-fat (1 percent), and reduced-fat (2 percent) milk ensures that the naturally beneficial fats and enzymes of milk are not available to the body.[24]

Drinking cow's milk without a sufficient level of the lactase enzyme can lead to lactose intolerance. Over fifty million adults in the United States are lactose intolerant, and an estimated 90 percent of Asian Americans and 75 percent of Native Americans and African Americans suffer from the condition, which can cause bloating, gas, cramps, vomiting, headaches, rashes, and asthma.[25]

In addition to lactose intolerance, the Physicians Committee for Responsible Medicine suggests that cancer, bone fractures, metabolic disorders, and heart diseases are also connected to increased consumption of dairy, and they recommend preventing these problems by eating a plant-based diet.[26]

Although American women consume tremendous amounts of calcium, much of it from milk products, their rates of osteoporosis are among the highest in the world. Chinese people consume half as much calcium (most of it from plant sources) and have a very low incidence of the bone disease. Medical studies indicate that rather than preventing osteoporosis, milk may actually increase women's risk of getting it. A study of more than seventy-seven thousand women ages thirty-four to fifty-nine found that increased milk consumption did not decrease the incidence of osteoporosis-related bone fractures.[27]

Milk and dairy products are not the only industrially produced foods that cause health issues. T. Colin Campbell, a professor of nutritional biochemistry at Cornell University, has pointed out the correlation between a high rate of protein consumption and the occurrence of life-threatening chronic diseases.[28]

Protein deficiency disease, or kwashiorkor, can be a problem in politically and racially created famines where people get less than five hundred calories from their daily intake of food. The same is not the case for the general well-fed public, yet they have been brainwashed into believing that because some protein is necessary for the body's good health, they must eat a lot of it every day. Eating too much animal protein, however, has been linked to the development of endometrial, pancreatic, and prostate cancer. It may also put a strain on the kidneys, causing them to compensate by leaching calcium from the bones.

Scientists at the National Institutes of Health have also found links between the consumption of industrially produced foods and an increase in the risk of prostate, breast, ovarian, uterine, and pancreatic cancers and brain tumors.[29] There are also links to an increased risk of arthritis, osteoporosis, hypertension, cardiovascular diseases, lymphoma, diabetes, obesity, food poisoning, and detectable levels of residual antibiotics and animal growth hormones in the blood. In addition, a gastrointestinal tract that is subjected to a daily intake of industrially produced foods begins to show a wide range of illnesses as well. Rates of esophageal, stomach, and colorectal cancers and ulcers are increasing. Leaky gut, gluten sensitivity, Crohn's disease, irritable bowel syndrome, bloating, indigestion, burping, acidity, gas, constipation, diarrhea, hemorrhoids, parasitic infestations, yeast overgrowth, malnutrition, allergies, indigestion, lethargy, and foggy brain have all become quite common. And if that wasn't enough, the consumption of highly processed foods has also been associated with the early onset of puberty, where girls as young as nine years old are reaching sexual maturity.[30]

In the end, extreme reliance on animal-based foods is considered unsustainable, and worldwide there is an emerging recognition of the role of plant-based foods for lowering and treating chronic diseases.[31]

IMPACT OF INDUSTRIALLY MANUFACTURED FOOD ON MENTAL/EMOTIONAL HEALTH

Besides the diseases expressed at physical levels, human society as a whole is suffering from psychological challenges as well. Even though we live in an age of unprecedented electronic connectivity via email, texts, sexts, Facebook, Snapchat, WhatsApp, Skype, FaceTime, and Tinder, people feel isolated, alone, scared, depressed, angry, irritable, unhappy, stressed, anxious, and full of previously unknown neurosis and psychosis. Our highly processed food is not only failing to feed our bodies, it is failing to feed our minds and souls as well.

The unprecedented level of involvement of the industrial manufacturing method in cultivation, harvest, and processing of plant-based foods and the industrialization of animal-based foods has ensured that we have no true, wholesome, deep connection to our food—or to each other. Because it is so removed from nature and her cycles and rhythms, our food has become unnatural, and our bodies and minds are paying a price for it. For these very reasons, it is crucial that we find ways to minimize the food-related problems that we are currently facing.

4

Principles of the Ayurvedic Reset Diet

How to Reboot Well-Being

This chapter will help you understand the principles of the Ayurvedic reset diet and why you should consider adopting it. In the upcoming sections, we will do the following:

- Explore the three main steps in the Ayurvedic reset diet and why we need them.
- Identify the main food groups and the many different eating styles they define.
- Learn how to combine food effectively and avoid viruddha ahara.
- Discover the roles that carbohydrates, fiber, protein, and fat play in our diet and how they are digested.

THE AYURVEDIC RESET DIET AND WHY WE NEED IT

As discussed in previous chapters, the advent of industrial food production and the year-round availability of all types of food has elicited a modern eating model that is enabling people to consume viruddha ahara, or foods that are mutually incompatible. Besides their reduced diversity and altered (destroyed) nutritional composition, these modern foods contain an excess of animal proteins and are packed heavily with salt, sugar, fats, antibiotics, antifungals, hormones, preservatives, colorants, and flavor enhancers as well as hundreds of other manmade chemicals. When these foods are combined and eaten in stressful conditions, year after year, with minimal amounts of calories being expended in exercising, the result is a direct increase in the number of discomforts and diseases that human beings experience. The body begins to rely heavily on the simple carbohydrates that are plentiful in modern foods for energy and heat, and the food from all the other groups is simply converted to fat and stored in the body. This lifestyle creates a fertile breeding ground for all the illnesses that compel us to rely on medications.

After digestion, the nutrients are absorbed in the small intestine. If the food contains very little or no fiber, then even though peristaltic movement keeps the chyme (pulp containing gastric juices and partly digested food) moving forward automatically, a lot of the chyme gets stuck in the folds (villi and microvilli) of the intestine, slowing down digestion and causing constipation. The chemical additives found in industrial foods are also absorbed into the body and enter the bloodstream. Antibiotics from these food sources disturb the gut bacteria, and excess soluble carbohydrates ferment in the colon and produce gas, causing distension and flatulence. Excessive distension can sometimes weaken the musculature so that hernias can protrude out.

Added to these issues is the simple fact that we have been eating three meals and a few snacks a day all of our lives—and our digestive system has been working constantly—even when we sleep—and has never had a chance to rest, to think (yes, there is something called "gut intelligence"), and to cleanse and repair itself. Over time, with nonstop performance and an overload of the wrong kind of food, the digestive system becomes sick and sluggish, and we are unable to get the nutritional benefits from the foods that we eat. At this point, though we are eating every day, we begin to show signs and symptoms of various illnesses that are directly connected with food, malnourishment, lifestyle, and stress. Our foods start a cascade of gene expression and biochemical reaction that creates an environment suitable for expression of diseases.

This is the reason we need to engage the Ayurvedic reset diet from time to time. It allows us to undo and reverse the effects of eating faulty food or wrongly combining different types of food, gives our gastrointestinal tract the much-needed free time to repair itself, and restores our sense of well-being and good health.

As I mentioned in the introduction, the Ayurvedic reset diet consists of three simple steps: (1) fasting on water only or water and herb teas only, (2) isolating food, and (3) mixing/combining foods from various food groups in a sensible way. In order to better understand the purpose for and reasoning behind these steps, it might be helpful to consider what modern science and Ayurveda have to say about them.

STEP 1: FASTING ON WATER ONLY OR WATER AND HERB TEAS ONLY

Fasting is a practice deeply ingrained in all old cultures of the world. Our hunter-gatherer ancestors knew very well that fasting from time to time helped them stay vigorous and active. They ate when food was available, and when it was not available for some reason, they did quite fine without it.

In Ayurveda, fasting is considered of prime importance in alleviating illness and bodily suffering from excessive food intake.[32] The Ayurvedic reset diet always begins with two days of fasting, during which you can drink water, as well as herbal teas with or without honey, but you abstain from eating solids. The reason for this is that fasting allows the body to obtain a much-needed rest from the continuous task of digesting food. During fasting, you can drink water and/or herbal tea to enable your body to flush itself out and turn on the cleanse switch to get rid of old, unwanted accumulations. Fasting on water/herbal tea also helps to wash out the oral cavity, clean up the dental biofilm, and improve oral hygiene. It also helps to flush out the overload of harmful germs from the gut.

It is estimated that the gut contains about ten times more bacteria than human cells. Most of these bacteria are useful and helpful. However, a lifelong habit of overeating wrongly mixed and industrially prepared foods that are low in fiber and high in refined carbohydrates, sugars, and "bad" fat, combined with insufficient water intake, causes serious gut dysbiosis (imbalance of the gut ecosystem), which leads to many chronic illnesses such as irritable bowel syndrome, obesity, diabetes, hypertension, cancer, autoimmune diseases, autism, hernias, and many other gastrointestinal illnesses.[33]

The mindful eating pattern that is established in the Ayurvedic reset diet facilitates reversal of the gut dysbiosis. Aided by fasting on water, and eating one type of food at a time, the harmful bacterial colonies are flushed out, and the useful bacteria are given an opportunity to recolonize the gut.

Though the knowledge and role of bacteria in health and disease is rather a nascent field of study that is still growing, the ancient science of Ayurveda recognizes *jeevanu* (life forms as small as an atom) just as the ancient schools of philosophy from India recognize the concept of *paramanu* (atoms). It stands to reason that very likely, the entire system of fasting as prescribed in Ayurveda was done to flush the body and get rid of everything that is harmful, including the harmful species of germs. Personally, I would not put it past the wit and wisdom of the ancient rishis who brought Ayurveda into existence.

MEMORY AND BLESSING OF WATER

An alternative medicine doctor from Japan, Masaru Emoto, began studying water in 1988.[34] Based on his experiments, he concluded that water responds to and remembers the energy it is exposed to and thus has the ability to memorize, copy, and transport information. In Ayurveda this is recognized through the practice of saying a blessing over water before drinking it.

Water molecules, their motions, and their alignment in space are affected by electromagnetic field energies. Their movements are not random. Everything creates vibrations and emits characteristic frequencies. These vibrations and frequencies are picked up by water molecules. They begin to retain the vibration and frequency they are exposed to and transmit these to the nearby water molecules until all of them vibrate at the same frequency. Molecules are very dynamic indeed. When electric charge is introduced into water, water molecules begin to reorient and realign themselves into clusters. Such clusters are bound by forces sufficient to generate further clusters, which are copies of the original cluster. These clusters are capable of carrying complex and subtle information as well as reproducing themselves and have enough energy to not be disrupted by random forces. It is also known that clusters of water molecules form coherent regions, and these can couple strongly with other fields of similar vibrations. Such coupling can harmonize the entire body of water. Coupling of coherent water clusters is not just a local but a global phenomenon, and coherent substances have the ability to transfer energy and information.[35]

The ability of water to memorize information is used in the application of water exposed to gemstones and colors for healing purposes. In relation to Homeopathy, which relies on the principle of "like cures like" through a pairing of vibrational frequencies of disease and remedy, Emoto's work supports the two fundamental methodologies used in preparation of homeopathic remedies—dilution and succussion. These processes enable the vibrational signature of the medicinal substance to be received by water and retained in water clusters. The more dilute the remedy, the more powerful it becomes, because the clusters of vibrational information are allowed to replicate and form new clusters with similar information.[36]

Because of its physicochemical nature, water gives us the power to create the change we want in ourselves. But note that water absorbs all frequencies it is exposed to . . . not just the positive ones. So it becomes imperative for us to live our lives wisely and cause the least amount of negativity, disruption, and damage by our thoughts, words, and actions to the environment we live in.

Old cultures and philosophies understood the power of water to absorb, retain, memorize, multiply, and transmit this message to those who seek, and they have accorded water a central position in all their ceremonies and celebrations. As water does have the ability to memorize the information it comes into contact with, we can expose it to the vibrations of our positive thoughts, intentions, words, and feelings in a mindful manner. During fasting, and even otherwise, by drinking water as a spiritual medicine that we can make for ourselves every day, we can create a positive and mindful impact on ourselves.

All we have to do is tune in and enjoy the blessings of water.

Physicochemical Properties of Water that Help Sustain All Life

- Water exists as solid (ice), liquid (water), and gas (vapor) at the temperatures and pressure normally found on Earth. The net water content of the Earth remains constant. Due to Earth's gravity, water vapors do not escape into outer space and disappear from the Earth's atmosphere.

- In its solid state, as ice, water molecules have large intermolecular spaces. This enables ice to be lighter than water and float above it and preserve life in ice-covered lakes and water bodies. Below a certain thickness of a sheet of ice, water remains as liquid at 4° C or 39° F, a temperature that sustains aquatic life.

- Water has a built-in self-purification process—while it changes from solid or liquid state into vapor form, it becomes pure because impurities do not vaporize and are left behind in the sediment.

- A stable proportion of saltwater to freshwater is maintained at 40:1, and this proportion keeps the density driven saltwater in the ocean and does not allow it to seep into the freshwater aquifers in the ground.

- As a universal solvent, water dissolves in itself almost everything that comes in contact with it and carries the solution to the ocean where marine life receives sustenance and nutrition from it.

All these physicochemical properties of water enable it to become indispensable for sustaining all life, including our own.[37]

IMPACT OF FASTING ON THE MOUTH

Fasting while drinking water not only helps you to remain well hydrated, it also flushes out the entire oral cavity. Without new food to get in the way, the movement of the water through the mouth allows small food particles from earlier meals to be cleaned out of the spaces between teeth and between the gums and teeth. This means that those particles are not providing food for the mouth bacteria and oral candida, preventing the bacterial action on food remnants that creates an acidic environment conducive to tooth enamel erosion. And when bad germs are not feasting and multiplying on remnants of food in the mouth, the beneficial oral germs can grow back and repopulate the oral cavity and help prevent dental diseases. The human mouth can host about six billion bacteria. Keeping them all in balance ensures better digestion of carbohydrates, which actually begins in the mouth. Reducing the bad bacteria also helps prevent bad breath.[38] All of these benefits are available to us simply from withholding food for a short duration and allowing water to flush out our mouth.

IMPACT OF FASTING ON THE BODY

While you are fasting, you are not providing any food to your body, so your digestive organs and glands do not have to work to digest food; they can rest. But resting for long is not in their nature. They are nonvoluntary organs, and nature has designed them to work around the clock. So when you do not give the digestive organs food to digest, they turn their attention to themselves and begin to shed unwanted tissues and old remnants and waste products. It is as if they clean themselves out with a scrubber and end up rejuvenated, revived, and repaired.

And when you drink plenty of water while you are fasting, it quickly passes through the digestive system in its downward journey and carries with it all the wastes that the digestive tract is shedding. It also literally washes and scrubs the surface of the stomach and all the other parts of the gastrointestinal tract and flushes the kidneys, bladder, and urinary tract as well.

Another action the body performs as soon as food is withheld during fasting is to begin to tap into stored glycogen for energy and heat. Glycogen gets stored in the liver as well as in the muscles and adipose tissue when excess food and more carbohydrates are consumed than are actually needed. Abstaining from food gives the body an opportunity to tap into its reserves of glycogen.[39] The store in the liver is easily accessible and is tapped first. When the liver reserve is used up, the body begins to metabolize the nutrients stored within the tissues. This process is known as autolysis. During moderate fasting autolysis is not a bad thing or something to be afraid of, as if organs are decomposing or the body is turning on itself by eating itself. In a controlled and conscious fasting program, autolysis is our friend.

Autophagy is yet another normal cellular process of self-correction that occurs in the body all the time even when we are not fasting, because this is how the body keeps itself free from injured and dead tissues. It is like routine housekeeping. The process of autophagy triggers a cascade of reactions within the cells, as the injured or dying cells and tissues are destroyed by their own enzymes and then enclosed in tiny sacs and delivered to the lysosomes (organelles present inside the cells) to be digested. Fasting enables the autophagy genes to be turned on and the process becomes even more efficient, speedier, and gives better results. In fact, the latest scientific research into the physiology of fasting is yielding amazing insight into what the body is capable of doing when food is withheld. In 2016 Japanese cell biologist Yoshinori

Ohsumi received a Nobel Prize in physiology and medicine for discovering that during fasting, cells simply turn on the autophagy gene. But rather than the injured or dying cells themselves being targeted, it's the unwanted, unnecessary, superfluous, and excess amounts of carbohydrates, proteins, and lipids that have been stored away in our cells from our days of (over)eating food that are packed up and delivered to the lysosomes. There they are digested by enzymes and broken down into simpler molecules that can be reused to provide fuel for energy and building blocks for the renewal of cellular structure.[40]

During a short period of fasting, the body also turns its attention to non-self cells, such as viruses, bacteria, and yeast that might be intruding on the cellular integrity of the body, and the same process of autophagy attacks these invaders and removes them from the system. When we are faced with various infections, the body turns on the autophagy gene and traps and digests the invading germs inside lysosomes, so the germs do not make us sick. Ayurvedic cures like abstaining from food during fevers and colds is an example of this principle in action.[41]

However, when our immunity is low, and our autophagy genes are defective or the physiological chain reaction that allows lysosomes to do autophagy is disrupted, then the germs are not cleared, and they can get the upper hand. Disruption in autophagy is now known to be linked with Parkinson's disease, type 2 diabetes, and other chronic illnesses like cancers.

Given all the above-mentioned benefits, it's no wonder that fasting is a prerequisite for the Ayurvedic reset diet. It is important to remember, however, that while short periods of fasting can be advantageous, fasting to an extreme and going without food for a very extended period of time—for example, when people with anorexia abstain from food and starve themselves—is a different matter. During such a severe lack of food, the process of autolysis begins to digest the essential tissues like muscles, which is obviously detrimental to the body. But you are not going to go that far when you practice the Ayurvedic reset diet, as it only requires a two-day fast with plenty of water to drink.

Water Fasting on Smart Vacations

It is interesting to note that the Ayurvedic prescription of engaging in water fasting has become a trend. People are spending prime dollars to go on what are called "smart vacations." They stay in fancy, high-priced hotels by the beach, but instead of gorging on opulent restaurant food and other gastronomic delights, they live on water alone with an occasional light plant-based meal.

It turns out that unlike regular tourists who run around their destination taking it all in, gorging on fancy, rich food, drinking alcohol in excess, and returning home exhausted and bloated, the water-only "smart vacationers" come back home rejuvenated. Besides giving their body rest and relaxation by being on a water-only fast, they are able to address some bothersome and serious health issues like obesity, indigestion, diabetes, high blood pressure, and depression and also cure themselves of colitis by engaging in a plant-based diet. A water-only fast, followed by a light diet of plant-based foods, sufficiently restricts smart vacationers' calorie consumption to allow their body to repair and reboot itself without medications. In addition to getting away from it all, smart vacationers on a water-only fast are able to improve their health.[42]

To recap, the benefits of fasting include the following:

- Cleansing of oral tissues, gums, and teeth from the addition of water and the absence of food
- Rest for the mouth from chewing
- Rest for the glands that service the digestive system
- Increase in energy because the digestive system is at rest
- Cleansing of the digestive tract by way of removal of old remnants in the small and large intestine, colon, and rectum
- Autolysis of unwanted, sick, and dying tissues

- Turning on of the autophagy gene so that autophagy happens at an accelerated pace during fasting
- Clearing of debris generated from autophagy
- Autophagy of excess stored fats in adipose tissues and organs
- Rejuvenation of healthy new tissues using the nutrients released from autophagy
- Removal of invading germs from the body

Now that you have a basic understanding of the reasons for and benefits of fasting with water, it's time to learn about isolating foods and avoiding faulty food combining.

STEP 2: ISOLATING FOODS AND AVOIDING INCOMPATIBLE FOOD COMBINATIONS

In this step, food ingredients are isolated in a sensible way, and only one type of food is eaten for a period of time. This allows the body to become adept at fully absorbing all the nutrients available in that one type of food, which, in turn, simplifies the process of digestion. This step is also a way of calling a halt to combining foods that don't work well together before recombining more compatible foods in a harmonious and productive way that better serves the body. This style of eating is also known as mono-diet.

To better grasp the need to isolate foods and avoid combining them inappropriately, it is necessary to have a basic understanding of the various food groups themselves as well as the many different eating styles they make up.

Food Groups and Eating Styles

The food groups listed below make up the essential sources of nourishment that the body needs to repair and regenerate itself and have enough energy for the activities of the daily life. All of the food groups have varying amounts of minerals, vitamins, micronutrients, enzymes, and phytochemicals (e.g., the dark, brilliant colors of leafy greens and fruits).

- Grains
- Legumes, nuts, and seeds
- Red meat and poultry
- Seafood and fish
- Eggs
- Dairy
- Vegetables
- Fruits
- Honey
- Fats (both plant and animal derived)

Many different eating styles are popular around the world, and they are determined by which of the various food groups mentioned above are eaten to obtain necessary nutrients. Listed in the table on page 61 are the various styles and the foods that define them.

The human body is designed to handle an omnivore eating style. While herbivores (e.g., horses, cows, and zebras) have flat teeth for grinding completely plant-based foods, and carnivores (e.g., dogs, lions, tigers) have very sharp, pointed canine teeth to tear at flesh, omnivores have both flat molars and sharp canines, enabling them to chew vegetables as well as animal flesh.

In ancient times, however, when the hunter-gatherers walked the earth, one's culture and the seasonal availability of food determined one's eating style. For example, people living in the polar circles could not grow and eat vegetables and fruits. They relied exclusively on hunting and eating animal-based foods for their survival. If a vegetarian went to live in a polar circle, he would not be able to stay alive unless he was willing to eat meat. However, nowadays, because of the global food trade and refrigerated transportation, any food is available anywhere and at any time. People can choose what to eat, depending on their personal needs, health, allergies, education, environmental awareness—and even personality!

EATING STYLES AND THEIR FOOD GROUPS

Eating Style	Grains	Legumes, Nuts & Seeds	Red Meat & Poultry	Seafood & Fish	Eggs	Dairy	Vegetables	Fruits	Honey	Plant-Based Fats	Animal-Based Fats
Omnivore	√	√	√	√	√	√	√	√	√	√	√
Paleolithic	X	√	√	√	√	X	√	√	Small amount	√	√
Pescatarian	√	√	X	√	√	√	√	√	√	√	Not lard
Reducetarian	√	√	√	√	√	√	√	√	√	√	√
(will eat a minimum amount of animal products)											
Lacto-vegetarian	√	√	X	X	X	√	√	√	√	√	Not lard
Lacto-ovo-vegetarian	√	√	X	X	√	√	√	√	√	√	Not lard
Vegan	√	√	X	X	X	X	√	√	X	√	X
Beegan	√	√	X	X	X	X	√	√	√	√	X
Gluten free	√	√	√	√	√	√	√	√	√	√	√
(will eat any of these foods as long as they don't contain gluten)											
Locavore	√	√	√	√	√	√	√	√	√	√	√
(will eat any of these foods if they come from within 100 miles)											
Rawtarian	√	√	√	√	√	√	√	√	√	√	√
(will eat any of these foods in raw form only)											
Fruitarian	X	X	X	X	X	X	X	√	X	X	X

In the sacred text Shrimad Bhagavad Gita, the food preferences of various personality types are described in terms of the three *gunas,* or qualities: *sattva* (harmony and balance), *rajas* (energy and action), and *tamas* (inertia and inactivity).

> The foods that promote life, vitality, strength, health, joy, and cheerfulness, which are sweet, soft, nourishing, and agreeable, are dear to the satviks (17:8).
>
> The foods that are bitter, sour, salty, very hot, pungent, harsh, and burning, producing pain, grief, and disease, are liked by the rajasik (17:9).
>
> The foods that are spoiled, tasteless, putrid, stale, refuse, and unclean is the food dear to the tamasik (17:10).

In addition to the gunas, Ayurveda also recognizes inherent differences in body type and how they relate to food choices. The three body types, or *doshas—kapha, vata,* and *pitta*—govern all aspects of the body, mind, and spirit. The beauty of these doshas is that a person is not exclusively ruled by just one. While a main dosha may predominate, the other two are still in the background and can affect a person as well.

Personally, I am one of those people who has always wondered which came first, the chicken or the egg. Are we born with specific dosha types that cause us to gravitate toward specific food groups or do we generate specific dosha patterns in our body based on the types of food we consume?

Logically, both of these scenarios are possible. Our birth and genetics determine the predispositions that we encounter in ourselves as we grow and become aware. At the same time, our food intake plays a huge role in turning on and off the various switches, so to speak, that bring about various dosha expressions and disease conditions. However, irrespective of the doshas we are born with, our life gives us many opportunities for making new choices, taking fresh initiatives, and traversing a path that enables us to obtain optimum wellness. The Ayurvedic reset diet is one such opportunity that can help us take charge of our life and transition to better health.

How Do We Avoid Combining Incompatible Foods?

Combining/mixing food means eating from more than one food group in a meal. Many or all of the food groups listed above are often eaten together in one meal. A typical example of this eating style is "casada," a typical platter of food served in Costa Rica. This platter contains rice, black beans, cheese, meat, eggs, cooked and raw vegetables, and fried plantain. It is an example of an omnivore eating style. Another example is a vegetarian platter from India. It can contain rice and wheat, a few different vegetables—steamed, stir-fried, curried with spices, or raw—at least a couple different legumes, nuts, cheese, yogurt, butter/ghee, honey, or fruits.

In contrast to these two widely popular eating styles that include or exclude several different food groups, the Ayurvedic reset diet focuses on eating only *one particular food at a time* and *in moderation*. Why should we undertake the Ayurvedic reset diet when we live in an age of opulence, where everything is available to us all the time? The simple answer is that it helps us undo the damage done to our body by excessive consumption of wrongly combined foods, or viruddha ahara.

What Is Viruddha Ahara?

In a mixed/combined meal, all food groups enter the gastrointestinal tract at the same time. But since the digestion of different food groups occurs at different times and locations, combining certain groups together at the same time can cause problems. Ayurveda offers instructions on how to avoid combining incompatible foods, or viruddha ahara, that are based on the knowledge about how food groups interact with each other. Ayurveda clearly describes the food groups that do not get along well and when eaten together can cause an interruption in the metabolism and absorption of nutrients. Paying attention to viruddha ahara is particularly important when trying to prevent or overcome chronic or acute illnesses. Ayurveda describes viruddha ahara as follows:

- Foods that are incompatible when combined (e.g., eating fish and milk in one meal)
- Food that has been wrongly processed (e.g., deep fried or burned food or heated honey)
- Food that is consumed in inappropriate amounts (e.g., combining equal amounts of salt and sugar or eating ten tablespoons of honey just because it is good for you)
- Food that is consumed at the wrong time of day (e.g., drinking coffee at night before bed or vinegar on an empty stomach)
- Food that is consumed in the wrong season (e.g., eating watermelon in the winter)
- Food that is consumed at the wrong temperature (e.g., drinking boiling hot coffee and simultaneously eating frozen berries and ice cream as dessert)

WHAT HAPPENS WHEN WE CONSUME INCOMPATIBLE FOOD, OR VIRUDDHA AHARA?

According to the Charaka Samhita, viruddha ahara eventually leads to morbidity, illness, and even death because it is not only bad for the digestive system, it also affects every other system of the body.[43] Eaten regularly, incompatible food combinations can also cause inflammation at a molecular level, which creates a number of metabolic disorders. Such ancient knowledge is sure to be of use to us as we look at the food we eat in the modern era.

The logical basis for avoiding viruddha ahara can be found in the study of the physiology and biochemistry of digestion of various food groups in the body. As per the tenets of Ayurveda, to avoid imbalance, proteins should not be combined with starches or carbohydrates and should be eaten at a different meal. Consuming these food groups together results in indigestion and the malabsorption of both groups, which prevents the body from extracting nutrients from either one. Eating proteins and starches together or proteins and sugars or acid fruits together hinders the action of ptyalin (an amylase enzyme in saliva that breaks down starch into maltose, a form of sugar[44]) and pepsin (a protease enzyme in the stomach that breaks down proteins), reducing the secretion of saliva and delaying digestion. If there is not enough amylase present in the mouth, starch will not be digested at all in the stomach and instead will clog up the intestine until the amylase in the small intestine can get to work on it.

Fats interfere with the secretion of digestive juices and reduce the amount of pepsin and hydrochloric acid in the stomach. As a result, digestion that happens in the stomach is slowed down considerably. Combining fats and carbohydrates has the same effect. So fats should be eaten in very small amounts when combined with protin- and carbohydrate-rich foods.

For a complete understanding of the benefits of the Ayurvedic reset diet, it is necessary to comprehend the physiology of digestion and the function of each of the various food groups. Because this understanding will also help you to make intelligent choices about what foods to eat together and what foods to eat separately, I have included detailed explanations in the sections below.

CARBOHYDRATES

Carbohydrates are obtained from grains, fruits, vegetables, and legumes and require an alkaline medium for digestion. As soon as saliva mixes with food in the chewing process, the digestion of carbohydrates begins.

During the process of chewing, food is exposed to the action of salivary enzyme, amylase. This enzyme immediately begins to break down complex carbohydrates, namely starches and glycogen, into simple carbohydrates, or glucose, galactose, and fructose.

Very soft foods, like white toast or mashed potatoes, do not have to be chewed for a long time, and they are swallowed as soon as they are mixed with saliva. Because the contact time between the food and the amylase in the mouth is not long enough for digestion to start right away, they reach the stomach in an undigested state. Coarse-skinned foods like celery, apples, or cucumbers, on the other hand, have to be chewed for a much longer time, allowing for the digestive process to begin, as it should, right in the mouth. The principles of Ayurveda recommend chewing food long enough for it to become the consistency of soft porridge.

As soon as chewed food, or bolus, reaches the stomach, gastric acids destroy the salivary amylase. Then the carbohydrates travel to the small intestine where they will be digested by pancreatic amylase. Complex carbohydrates are known as polysaccharides. Pancreatic amylase converts these polysaccharides into simple carbohydrates, which are metabolized in the liver. From here, the simple carbohydrates go to peripheral tissues and the bloodstream. Any carbohydrates that are not immediately used are converted into glycogen and stored in liver and muscles.[45]

Fiber

Fiber—both soluble and insoluble—is also a carbohydrate. Soluble fiber absorbs and dissolves in water. It turns into a gelatinous mass and reaches the large intestine where it ferments, produces gas, and provides nutrients to the gut bacteria. Insoluble fiber is not affected by digestive enzymes. It reaches the colon unchanged and contributes to the formation of the stool.[46]

Recently, *Lancet,* a medical journal of high repute, published a review of 243 studies on fiber. According to the studies, people who eat fiber-rich foods cut their risk of heart disease, stroke, hypertension, type-2 diabetes, and cancer by 15 to 30 percent. The best sources of fiber are fruits and vegetables, whole grains, nuts, legumes, and seeds. Fiber-rich foods take longer to chew and digest, so people feel fuller more quickly and remain full for a longer time, so they tend to eat less and do not need to eat as frequently. A high-fiber diet enables the beneficial bacteria in the gut to help in the maturation process of the immune system and thus reduces the risk of conditions such as colon cancer. Fiber-rich foods also help to slow down the release and absorption of glucose, so blood-sugar levels do not go up and down as quickly as they do with refined foods without fiber. Getting fiber from whole foods is better than taking it in supplemental form because in addition to fiber, whole foods also contain loads of other micronutrients, vitamins, and enzymes.[47]

Functions of Carbohydrates

- Provide a rapid source of energy and heat
- Reduce the need for protein to provide energy and heat
- Store energy for when food becomes scarce (after the necessary glycogen has been stored away, any excess carbohydrates turn into fat and stay under the skin to be used as needed)

PROTEINS

Proteins are obtained from meats, fish, seafood, dairy, legumes, and nuts. Protein digestion requires an acid medium, and it occurs in the stomach and duodenum where three main enzymes break down proteins into peptides. Further down in the small intestine, these peptides break down into amino acids and are absorbed into the bloodstream to be used for the growth and repair of the body. Excess protein is converted into fat and stored in adipose tissues, and the nitrogen part of protein is converted into urea and excreted via kidneys.[48]

Functions of Protein

- Growth and repair of tissues
- Synthesize enzymes, globulins, and hormones
- Provide energy

Providing energy is a secondary function of proteins. As long as there are enough carbohydrates available, protein is not used for making energy. In fact, the presence of refined carbohydrates without fiber in a meal directly interferes with the energy-providing function of proteins and helps convert excess protein into fat. Excess protein also puts an extra load on the kidneys.

FATS

the Fats are obtained from animal and vegetable sources. Saturated fats from milk, butter, ghee, cheese, lard, meat, and fish are converted into "bad," low-density cholesterol. Unsaturated fats from fish, nuts, and vegetable oils help reduce low-density cholesterol and increase the good, high-density cholesterol.49 Fats are digested in the small intestine by bile from the liver and lipase enzymes from the pancreas.

Functions of Fats

- Provide energy and heat
- Support cellular structure
- Help transport fat soluble vitamins A, D, E, and K
- Maintain nerve structures
- Make cholesterol and hormones

Though fats do provide energy and heat, again, when excess carbohydrates are consumed along with fat, then the carbohydrates do the job of providing heat and energy and do not give fats a chance to do so. As a result, any dietary fat that does not get used to perform the functions listed above, including heat and energy production, ends up being stored in the adipose tissues and around internal organs including the liver.[50] Subcutaneous fat is stored mainly in the arms and legs, but visceral fat is stored around abdominal organs. Visceral fat accumulation is a precursor of several lifestyle-related diseases such as hypertension, type 2 diabetes, glucose intolerance, heart disease, and various cancers.

Fat is essential to the body. When fat—in moderation and of the right kind—enters the intestine along with carbohydrates and proteins, it helps us feel full. Modern non- or low-fat versions of dairy products and any other food are not desirable.[51] Loss of fat leads to loss of taste, and to make up for it, sugar—a simple carbohydrate—is added. This extra sugar interferes with the body's use of proteins and fats for energy and heat, and as mentioned above, any unused proteins and fats, or carbohydrates for that matter, all get converted into fat and are stored in the body. In trying to avoid fat, we actually end up accumulating more of it in our body. Non-fat and low-fat foods such as yogurt actually backfire. When we eat them, we are deprived of a healthy intake of fat, and a lack of fat means the body does not get the satiety signal, so we tend to eat more.

Artificial butters and margarine are also found to be quite harmful.[52] The best option is to stick with natural sources of dairy fat and rely on unrefined and raw oils from vegetable sources, such as coconuts, olives, sesame seeds, peanuts, almonds, mustard, flax, hemp, avocados, and so on. It is good to use all types of fat sparingly.

The Risks of Reheating Fats

Ayurveda maintains that fats and oils should not be reheated. Current science can easily confirm that reheating oil leads to oxidation, and oxidized oils cause the formation of free radicals, or unstable atoms, in the body, which can lead to inflammation. Oxidative rancidity occurs when fatty acids are exposed to oxygen in the presence of heat or light, resulting in the formation of hydroperoxide compounds, which are converted to aldehyde molecules. These molecules are toxic and cause oxidative stress in the cells and are likely to increase the risk of degenerative illness and atherosclerotic disease. Overheated and oxidized fats also interfere with fat-soluble vitamins A and E.

The degree of saturation in oil is an important factor in determining the quality of cooking oils. Unsaturated fatty acids are more susceptible to oxidation than saturated fatty acids, and for this reason they are a source of free radicals. A recent study found that a toxin called 4-hydroxy-trans-2-nonenal (HNE) forms when unsaturated fatty acids (oils) from vegetable sources like corn, soybean, and sunflower are reheated. The consumption of foods containing HNE from cooking oils has been associated with an increased risk of cardiovascular disease, stroke, Parkinson's disease, Alzheimer's disease, Huntington's disease, various liver disorders, and cancer.[53] Because of these dangers, the excess use of fats and oils and the consumption of deep-fried foods and baked goods made with unhealthy fats are considered viruddha ahara and contraindicated in the Ayurvedic reset diet.

VITAMINS

Both fat-soluble (A, D, E, and K) and water-soluble (B complex and C) vitamins are directly absorbed into the body and used as micronutrients. Vitamin D, pyridoxine, niacin, and biotin are stable, but all the others are destroyed through cooking and exposure to light, air, water, and strong acids and alkalis.[54] This is the reason that rawtarians eat only those foods that can be eaten completely raw.

STEP 3: MIXING/COMBINING FOODS FROM VARIOUS FOOD GROUPS IN A SENSIBLE WAY

When we eventually return to mixing and combining foods, the body has been rebooted, rejuvenated, and retrained by the first two steps in the Ayurvedic reset diet, and it is now able to adjust to the availability of various nutrients *that are compatible with each other.* The invigorated digestive system is able to absorb these multiple nutrients for the growth and repair of the body.

Having learned about viruddha ahara, you can now be very keen and mindful about what type of food you will allow into your body. After all, the real estate in your stomach is very precious. You cannot fill it up with "garbage" forms of food. Once you have completed the fasting and isolating foods steps, your body will have worked hard to repair and rejuvenate itself and had the opportunity to tap into its glycogen and fat reserves as well as seek out unwanted tissues from which to extract nutrients.

The plan laid out in the Ayurvedic reset diet step 3, when you get to eat a wide variety of food after two weeks of eating vegetables only and two weeks of eating fruits only, is designed with consideration of what foods are okay to mix and how much time various foods take to digest and clear out of the stomach. When you start mixing food, you are back to receiving nutrients from a wide variety of sources, but the mixing is done so that the digestive system has enough time to deal with the various food groups because they are eaten in a sensible order.

In the Ayurvedic reset diet, the sequence of eating various foods is such that carbohydrates and proteins are not all mixed up in the intestine, and therefore, food is not fermenting and producing volumes of gas. You get to eat from all the food groups—fruits, vegetables, grains, legumes, meat, seafood, eggs, and dairy—but you are eating *from just one food group at any time.*

As shown above, various food groups need different amounts of time for digestion. When only one food group is eaten at a time, the body does not have to struggle to digest carbohydrates, fats, proteins, and fiber all at once. The Ayurvedic reset diet allows your body to completely digest and then extract all the nutrients from each food group because only one type of food is passing through the intestines in any given time, so even though you get to eat from all of the food groups, your digestive system remains relaxed and does not experience food fermentation in the intestines.

The Ayurvedic reset diet is based on the idea that the foods that are easiest to digest are eaten at breakfast, giving you a burst of good energy to start your day. For this reason, breakfast comprises whole fruits, nuts, and seeds.

Five to six hours later, you eat a lunch of carbohydrates consisting of grains, vegetables, and salads. Your body has to work a bit harder to digest this meal than it did breakfast, but since all the ingredients are plant-based, they will be digested within six hours, and the contents of your stomach will clear out. Carbohydrates also provide a quick source of energy and heat. Eating foods rich in carbohydrates gives the body sufficient energy during the daytime because your vital energy is not bogged down with heavy-to-digest food like meat or legumes. And since you remain physically active during the day, the easily available energy from carbohydrates is used up in your day-to-day activities and, provided you do not eat in excess, no additional glucose needs to be converted to glycogen and stored away in the liver for later use.

Six hours later, in the evening, you sit down to a dinner of legumes or meat. Eating these protein-rich, hard-to-digest foods separately from carbohydrate sources and at night when the body is at rest gives them sufficient time to digest. Also, since you do not eat any fruits, vegetables, or grains in this meal, these sources of carbohydrates are not fermenting in your intestine while it is trying to digest the meats and legumes.

Eating Less Red Meat
May Help You Live Longer

Though vegetarian and vegan styles of eating are on the rise, there is a significant percentage of the global population that relies heavily on meat and animal-based food for their protein. It is not necessary for everyone to become vegetarian or vegan. If you want to continue eating animal-based food, that is your choice. However, please bear in mind a study done by Dr. Frank Hu of Harvard University that concluded that eating less red meat (beef, lamb, etc.) helps you live longer. Dr. Hu and his team followed the eating habits of fifty-four thousand women and twenty-eight thousand men from thirty to seventy-five years of age, for eight years. They found that when participants increased their red meat intake by half a serving a day—the equivalent of one-and-a-half slices of roast beef—their risk of an early death rose by 10 percent. The consumption of an extra half a serving of processed meats like bacon and sausage increased the risk of an early death by 13 percent. In contrast, participants who cut down their consumption of red meat also had a reduction in their rate of premature death. When participants ate fish instead of a daily serving of unprocessed or processed red meat, their risk of premature death fell by 17 to 25 percent. The consumption of chicken and protein from plant-based sources gave a comparable result. It would be wise, therefore, to avoid or reduce red meat even if going vegan or vegetarian is not your cup of tea.

The Ayurvedic reset diet allows us to *undo and reverse* the deleterious effects of viruddha ahara and paves the way for a healthier style of eating. I routinely recommend it, along with modifications, tips, and healthy recipes, to my clients when they come for a consultation. Several of my clients who have practiced this diet have reported optimum wellness and a noticeable reduction in their health complaints.

In the next chapter we will explore a number of actions you can take to properly prepare for implementing this diet into your life.

5

Preparing for the Ayurvedic Reset Diet

Actions to Take before You Begin

You have so far gathered every bit of background information about what the Ayurvedic reset diet is and why there is a need for practicing it. Now you are ready to take the concrete and practical actions that will enable you to actually engage in this unique and life-enhancing, life-affirming activity.

The whole enterprise begins with saying goodbye to your old habits, doubts, and excuses. (I agree, this is hard to do, and I have struggled with it myself.) Then it's time to purge the kitchen cabinets of unnecessary and harmful foods to make room for more health-promoting, wholesome, and real foods. Since the Ayurvedic reset diet requires that you eat just one type of simple food in moderation for a period of time, it implies that there will be a cleaning up of your food habits as well as your digestive system. I will make suggestions on which food items you need to get rid of and recommendations on what new foods to shop for and where.

Once the cabinets have been cleaned out and the unhealthy foods have been discarded, you will discover how to cleanse yourself, both inside and out, and how to keep diversions out of your dining room and create a clean, pleasing space for enjoying your food. Finally, you will learn how to satisfy all five of your senses by eating with your hands.

ACTION 1: BANISH DOUBTS AND EXCUSES

Now that the much-awaited time has come to take some concrete action to prepare for this life-changing activity, the law of inertia will most likely kick in and many, many reasons why you cannot practice the Ayurvedic reset diet will come up in your mind. You will want to remain stuck to your old habits and routines. You might think you are too busy, too tired, too sick, or too hungry, or simply too disorganized. You might consider yourself young and healthy enough not to need a new diet. You may also have tried a few different diets where the results fell short of your expectations, or you know that most diets floating around in the market are trying to sell something to you.

Next, doubts about the process itself will come up. Is it really good for you? Why choose this diet instead of any other available on the market? You might also wonder if your body will get enough nutrition when you're on the Ayurvedic reset diet. How will you cope with hunger? How will you cope with the temptation to drop the diet and eat whatever you want because plenty of food is available?

You might also think that you do not have sufficient willpower to stick with a discipline and routine for any stretch of time, or if you do stick with the routine, you might feel that your personal freedom is hindered. You may also feel that if you do this Ayurvedic reset diet for yourself, by yourself, it means that you are focusing on yourself too much and not giving enough attention to your family. You might even do a little calculation and come up with a number that says organic foods (recommended in general and particularly during the Ayurvedic reset diet) are more expensive than regular foods and that you do not want to be selfish and spend all that money on yourself.

If so, you're not alone. I have been recommending the Ayurvedic reset diet to my clients since starting my practice in 2008. Let me give you a summary of the responses I have gotten. Some people—yes, there are quite a few of them—hold on to the method, the technique, with all their might. Come what may, they see it through and complete the full process. They are careful to cross all the t's and dot all the i's, and their tenacity and determination amaze me.

Apart from these dedicated individuals, I have also met several innovator types who have liberally and literally played with the idea, picked the part of the program that they liked, and then followed that part from time to time. Some have skipped the first two days when you can take water only followed by alternating water and herbal teas only, and gone straight to the fruits-only or vegetables-only weeks. Here are some of the reasons they gave:

"I am healthy enough, why should I fast?"

"Oh! I never drink water. I am not the thirsty type."

"I get nauseous when I drink water. Water is so bland!"

"Honey is not for me . . . I am vegan."

"I detest herbal teas . . . if I must have tea, I will go for the real stuff—full-blast caffeinated black tea with cream and sugar. Why should I subject myself to fake tea?"

Others want to skip the fruits-only or vegetables-only week saying:

"I do not like fruits. The sweet taste puts me off."

"I get too gassy."

"Just the thought of eating cold or room-temperature fruit day in and day out bores me."

"Yuck! Vegetables are yuck!"

"I eat tomato ketchup and that is my vegetable."

"Anything that is not peeled, white, soft, buttered, and puréed [i.e., mashed potato] is not worth eating."

"Well, cows eat grass, and I eat cows, so I get the essence of grass from that."

"I am very alternative minded and green-conscious, do not mistake me, please, but that doesn't mean I will eat vegetables."

The bottom line is, people can be very creative, innovative, clever, and resourceful when they have to come up with a reason why they cannot do something. That's okay; it's human nature. There is after all no such thing as one size fits all. That concept works for the retail giants who want to push cheap stuff made in the sweatshops to consumers of all ages and sizes and make a fast buck. But as far as anything to do with human nature and wellness is concerned, people are very different; they are not churned out in cookie factories. A person's likes, dislikes, desires, aversions all come into play as they make choices and decisions for themselves.

But I will ask you now to weigh your health on one side and all the questions, doubts, and excuses on the other side to see which is heavier, i.e., more important to you. In my view, those thoughts that are holding you back have a place in your life only as long as you do not decide to take charge of your own wellness. Once you truly begin to care for your health and see that it is the most precious thing you have in your life, then you will find enough determination and willpower to begin and complete the Ayurvedic reset diet successfully and see for yourself what it can do for your well-being. Intentions are powerful: Make a commitment to wellness, set your intention to give the Ayurvedic reset diet a try, and heal yourself.

ACTION 2: CLEAN OUT THE CABINETS

Cleaning out the external world of your kitchen cabinets, fridge, freezer, and pantry is an essential part of starting your Ayurvedic reset diet, which is going to focus on the inner cleaning of your gastrointestinal system. Perhaps up until now you have filled your pantry, freezer, and refrigerator with food choices based on what you feel like eating, what is inexpensive, or what is readily available in supermarkets. When you make a commitment to the Ayurvedic reset diet, however, you will be shopping with a different mindset and thus most likely choosing different foods. But before your next shopping expedition, you need to clean out the unnecessary items from your kitchen and pantry to make room for the new foods.

A Note about Shopping Bags

Numerous cities in the United States have banned plastic grocery bags that do not biodegrade and end up polluting the entire eco-system. Since you are embarking on an inner and external cleaning process, this may be a good time to say goodbye to single-use plastic grocery bags and use either cloth bags or biodegradable bags made from cornstarch. Every plastic bag that is not used is a bag that does not end up in the landfill or float in the ocean for the next one thousand years.

WHAT SHOULD COME OUT OF THE FRIDGE, FREEZER, AND PANTRY?

The following is a list of items that should be removed from your refrigerator, freezer, cupboards, and pantry before you start the Ayurvedic reset diet:

- Industrially prepared fruit juices, jams, jellies, and dried fruits that are chemically colored and contain a high amount of added sugars
- Sugar and artificial sweeteners including agave nectar, aspartame, stevia, and Splenda
- Sodas and soft drinks, including "diet" versions
- Vodka, wine, beer, and alcohol
- Flour, pastas, breads, and baked goods made from refined wheat flour

- White rice and all products made with refined white rice flour
- Saturated hydrogenated fats, artificial cheese, artificial burgers, and artificial hotdogs, all of which are vegan/vegetarian options that are processed to look and taste like cheese or meat by using numerous chemical processes
- Processed meats like salami, hot dogs, and meatballs
- Artificially or industrially prepared and packaged foods, frozen foods, snacks, etc.
- Store-bought tortillas, empanadas, cakes, desserts, ice cream, and cookies, as well as milk chocolate
- Anything that contains trans fats

When you read through this list, you will see that processed and sugary foods are the target. And rightly so, as studies keep coming out that highlight the dangers of these types of foods. Take, for example, fruit juices. The label on the bottle might declare that it contains the purest fresh juice from fruits. However, pure or not, it is just as dangerous as soda with added sugar and will invariably lead to obesity. Sugary beverages, including fruit juices, increase insulin resistance and that leads to cardiovascular diseases. Similarly, juices and beverages sweetened with a high concentration of fructose cause weight gain around the middle.

By eliminating the foods listed above, you will easily be able to shave off anywhere from three hundred to five hundred calories from your meals. This is the number of calories that are present in a large bagel, a couple of chocolate chip cookies, a bag of chips, or a cup of ice cream. These innocent-looking foods of our daily life are calorie bombs that we drop mindlessly into our stomach.

A study done by William Kraus of Duke University was reported in the *New York Times*. Apparently healthy men and women from the ages of twenty-one to fifty were observed for two years. They had dropped their daily caloric intake 12 to 25 percent, about three hundred calories or more. The benefit of such a small reduction was significant.

They lost body weight as well as accumulated fat; their blood pressure, blood sugar, and cholesterol levels improved; and they experienced less inflammation. Dr. Kraus's team concluded that such improvements were not just the result of weight loss but also of the reduction in calorie intake and that similar results were hard to come by even when five different drugs were prescribed to address weight, sugar, cholesterol, and inflammation.[55]

Along the same lines, another study by researchers at the National Institutes of Health found that when people are given ultra-processed foods, they tend to eat faster and easily consume an additional five hundred calories a day because ultra-processed foods are easier to eat, cheaper, and designed to create a sense of dependence on them.[56]

Another study that comes to mind was conducted by Dr. Farokh Master, a homeopath in India. His study/observation points out that insulin resistance and higher blood glucose levels together have a role in eliciting cancer.[57]

The foods that I am suggesting you remove from your kitchen come under the banner of "comfort food." The world's best-known comfort food—cookies—are made using a ton of sugar, wheat flour, and fat. Anyone who has indulged in comfort foods is aware that once you start eating them, it is rather difficult to stop. The reason for this is because while they are offering us "comfort," they are also creating habit and dependency. We begin to get addicted to the taste and comfort level that the act of eating the food brings us. Then, instead of eating to live, we begin to live to eat. Our desire and need for comfort make us eat like a robot—eat, eat, eat, and eat some more without missing a single meal or snack. We have developed the habit of eating nonstop, and we have resigned to getting sick from our food.

Omitting the foods listed above will help you steer away from comfort foods that spike your blood sugar and increase your fat, cholesterol, and weight. By taking the bold move of avoiding these foods, you are choosing to ignore the whispers that can sidetrack you from your mission of practicing the Ayurvedic reset diet.

As you read further, you will see that although some foods have been omitted, there is a very large variety of foods that you are given the freedom to indulge in that will promote well-being. If you are expecting to experience unbearable hunger, low energy, starvation, deprivation, and scarcity while practicing the Ayurvedic reset diet, you will truly have to look elsewhere.

When you get rid of the items listed above, you might think you are wasting your hard-earned money and throwing useful things away. However, because you are committed to the Ayurvedic reset diet, they are not useful to you right now and will only serve as a distraction. It would be best to get rid of them.

ACTION 3: SHOP FOR HEALTHIER FOOD

Shopping for healthier, more natural food is an investment in and a positive step toward your well-being and another creative and enjoyable step toward your goal of practicing the Ayurvedic reset diet. Instead of going back to the regular supermarket that has sold you industrially grown junk food for years, locate a health food store nearby. Get a membership if it ensures some additional discounts and provides information on the arrival of fresh foods. Most health-food stores give discounts to people over sixty-five years of age and often even have parking spaces reserved for seniors!

If you are lucky enough to locate a farmers market that sells locally grown, organic foods, these can be the freshest, best foods available to you. Better yet, you can grow your own organic lettuce, microgreens, carrots, kale, scallions, edible herbs, tomatoes, lemons, and ginger in gardens in your yard or in containers on a patio or indoors if you live in a city.[58] These tiny crops will be as local as you can get . . . right out of your own garden or pot and grown by your own hands.

If shopping more frequently is possible at all, it is highly recommended. Multiple outings to the farmers market or health food store each week give you a reason to get dressed and get out of the house, move, mingle with people, socialize, become friendly with the farmers, and learn about their farming practices as well as allow you to get fresher foods. Although their numbers are rising steadily, organic farmers are still few and far between. When you purchase directly from a farmer and show appreciation for the work they do to make organic food items available to you, they get more inspired to stick with organic farming.

It is especially beneficial to shop for produce two or three times every week. Most of these items will have to be refrigerated if you keep them long and therefore, it is good to buy them in small quantities and purchase more as and when you need per the meal plan. Refrigerated fruits and vegetables stay good a bit longer, but refrigeration and freezing deteriorates micronutrients, particularly water-soluble vitamins, and you are left with only fiber, carbohydrates, and minerals. This is also why local is best, as transport over long distances requires refrigeration and freezing.

Organic, Locally Grown Food

Having read about the atrocities that animals are subjected to and the manner in which the environment is destroyed in industrial agriculture and animal husbandry, any person who wants good health for herself and the planet we live on will lean toward organically grown food. Organic farmers do not support using commercial/industrial pesticides, herbicides, fertilizers, weed killers, fungicides, or genetically engineered grains, fruits, vegetables, or meats. Because organic growing processes are free of chemicals, they do not harm the environment, the oceans, or our bodies the way industrial foods do. They are as much "back to nature" as the methods of our hunter-gatherer ancestors in prehistoric times.

In addition to organically grown plants, there are free-range systems where animals are housed in barns or aviaries but also have access to an outside range with vegetation. In the European Union, free-range birds must have constant daytime access to at least 4 square meters (about 43 square feet) of outside space. In the United States, there are no specified requirements for space and duration of time to qualify as "free-range," so know your labels! Organic farms in the European Union certified by the Soil Association have even broader outdoor and indoor space requirements as well. In the United States there are general living condition guidelines for the organic label but no specific space requirements. In both places, in organic meat and milk production, growth hormones and antibiotics are not used to fatten animals and food sources must be organic—for example, beef cows are not given asbestos to eat and chickens are not fed manure as often occurs on industrial farms. There are also stricter guidelines around the treatment of animals for organically certified food, but again, these can be vague, so know your certifications and labels.

Although organic foods might seem more expensive on the surface, their quality is so far superior to that of conventional foods that the cost is easily justified. Since the nutrients per serving obtained from organic foods are far higher than those obtained from conventional foods, you end up paying many times over to get the same amount of nutrients from conventional foods. And because you do not get the nutrients you need for good health from your conventional foods, you end up eating a lot more in search of those nutrients than your body needs, which may lead to unwanted weight gain and other health issues. You could also wind up spending a lot more money for nutritional supplements to make up for those lost nutrients. And in general, both the added chemicals and the lack of nutrients in the industrial food cause you to be sick more often and, in turn, spend more money on medical bills. The end result of purchasing and consuming industrial foods is that you do not get the nutrients nature is providing you for free by way of whole, unprocessed foods, you get sick, and you end up spending more money in the long run. Any way you look at it, organic foods are better for your conscience, better for your health, and better for the planet.

Although it would be beneficial for all organic foods to be seasonal, nowadays, they simply aren't. Industrialization has moved us too far from nature. Even the best and strictest organic superstores in the

United States now carry summer fruits and vegetables in the winter and winter fruits and vegetables in the summer. Organic foods grown in other countries with better growing climates are flown in and trucked to organic supermarkets. Organic meats of all kinds are also available throughout the year. So seasonality is gone from even the organic shelves of the supermarkets. Even with some loss of nutrients that happens from transport and refrigeration, organic foods still come to you without the additional burden of toxic, manmade pesticides, herbicides, fertilizers, antifungals, antibiotics, preservatives, antifreeze chemicals, artificial colors, growth hormones, or artificial flavors. Organic foods are not genetically engineered. By that count, it is still much preferable to eat organic foods even nonlocally or out of season than to make up for the loss of vitamins by taking nutritional supplements.

Eating Seasonally in Northern Climates

If you live in the North America, looking for *fresh* mangos will be a waste of time, as these have been grown thousands of miles away in hot climates, harvested when still unripe, and transported by ships, planes, trains, and trucks to your market. How fresh can they be even if the label says they are organic? Take another example: Watermelons are available in northern supermarkets almost throughout the year and so are apples. But it is well-known that watermelon is a summer fruit and an apple is a colder weather fruit. So we make a choice; we eat watermelon in the summer and apples in the winter. Similarly, squashes, pumpkins, and root vegetables of all types could be stored in cellars to help get us through winter months and these vegetables might be a better winter choice in a New England supermarket.

A good place to get food that you know is seasonal is a local farmers market, farm stand, or farm store. If you're lucky enough to have one nearby that operates year-round, you will see how the kinds and quantity of fruit and vegetable options change with the seasons.

However, in your search for organic foods, do not be fooled by the words on the label that say "All natural" or "Grown without the use of additional chemicals." Industrial manufacturers have learned that consumers are attracted to the word *natural,* so they now use this word indiscriminately and "grown without the use of additional chemicals" implies that at least some chemicals were used. When you spend your money on organic goods, look for the "USDA organic" label.

Locally grown but not certified organic versus certified organic from hundreds or thousands of miles away—what type of produce and groceries are best? There are arguments in favor of both. Certified organic food flown in from afar creates a ton of pollution (think transportation) and people are put off by that. They want to get locally grown food from within a 100-mile radius. The recent farm-to-table movement is a reflection of the desire of people for locally grown food. The intention of eating locally grown food is indeed good, if the local food is organic but does not carry the third-party certification. The small-scale local farmers might practice all procedures for raising an organic crop but do not have the funds for the bureaucratic process of obtaining a third-party certification. However, if local growers are using nasty chemicals for their agriculture, then of course we are better off buying certified organic items that are not local. The idea is that as best as we can, we have to stay away from the nasty, toxic stuff that is used in growing food.

Also, as you become more aware of what to buy, make sure you stay away from organic junk foods. These are very attractively packaged with beautiful photographs of food on the outside and a label tagging every ingredient with the word *organic.* Although the ingredients may technically be organic, they can be made from refined flour and other ingredients as well as be deep fried. They might be full of sugars and salts to make them taste "better," especially in fat-free versions. Or they might even include protein isolates, which are made in a highly industrialized process and require a ton of chemicals that your body does not need. Although they are organic, they are essentially no better than commonly available junk foods.

Shopping for Nonperishable Items

The items listed below do not have to be refrigerated or frozen, and they keep well for a long time if stored properly in airtight containers. You can shop for smaller quantities or stock up on larger amounts depending on your schedule, finances, and location. It is important to find organic, unprocessed versions of these foods (note that organic does not necessarily indicate unprocessed). Here are two examples of why: Vitamin B-complex is found in the brown skin of rice. Magnesium is found in the red-purple skin of peanuts. But in the manufacturing process, even if rice and peanuts are organically grown, their brown skins are removed, and essentially, these valuable nutrients are thrown out as by-products and wastes. The lifelong consumption of even organic white rice and peanuts without skins means that you have never received the gift of these nutrients from nature. Over the years, you start developing some nerve-related problems, and you get a prescription for B-complex tablets or injections and magnesium capsules—unnecessary and avoidable issues and expenses.

Grains: Barley, buckwheat, millet, quinoa, rye, unpolished black or brown wild rice with bran, and whole grain oats.

Honey: This should be natural, locally produced, raw, unrefined, and unpasteurized. Local honey simply means that the honeybees have had the great fortune of visiting cultivated or wild flowers for collecting nectar. This is very important because these flowers grow in your region. Honey made from their nectar works like a natural antibiotic for handling infections like colds, skin rashes, mouth sores, and sore throats. Honey naturally contains some hydrogen peroxide, which helps to keep localized infections in check. Even type 2 diabetics can eat honey in very small amounts. Honey is the oldest known Ayurvedic remedy. Pasteurized, refined honey made in China—even if the label says it is organic—is not as good for you as locally and noncommercially made honey. Industrially and commercially produced honey is made by giving the bees sugar syrup instead of allowing them to collect nectar from wildflowers. There is nothing natural about this industrial honey.[59]

Legumes: Beans, dals, and pulses are all included in the group legumes. Most can be cooked and eaten with the skin so that more fiber, plant-based pigments, and minerals can be obtained. Adzuki beans, anasazi beans, black beans, black-eyed peas, chickpeas (garbanzo beans and Bengal grams),* cranberry beans, French lentils,* fava beans, kidney beans, lima beans, Mexican red beans, mung beans (whole* and split), navy beans, red lentils (masoor dal),* peas (including dried whole* and split), pinto beans, soy beans, tuvar dal (pigeon pea), urad dal (split and whole), white beans, and any other legume that you can find in the farmers market. Buy beans with their skin on. Legumes are also considered to be healthier proteins.[60]

Nuts: Almonds, Brazil nuts, cashews, chestnuts, hazelnuts, macadamias, pecans, peanuts (technically considered a legume, but eaten as a nut for our purposes), pistachios, and walnuts. Some nuts have a skin that can be peeled. For example, you can remove the reddish-purple skin found on peanuts after you take the peanuts out of the shell. Similarly, you can get almonds without the thin brown skin. However, the edible skin of various nuts and seeds contain a rich supply of minerals, fiber, and phytonutrients. Discarding the skin means we are throwing away those nutrients, and the nuts become simply a source of protein and fat.

All these nuts can be eaten raw, so you need not buy roasted or fried nuts that are coated with sugar or salt. Though nut butters such as peanut butter, almond butter, and cashew butter are popular, they can go "stale" when the oil gets oxidized, and they do not have the nutritional benefit of the nuts' skin. Like legumes, nuts are considered healthier proteins. Unlike red meats, which contain a lot of saturated fats, the proteins available in nuts come with a natural amount of unsaturated

---

*Beans, pulses, and dals marked with an * can be very easily germinated at home. After sprouting, they can be eaten raw, and are very easy to digest.

fats. These healthy fats can reverse the problems created by overconsumption of red meat and saturated fats.[61]

Oils: Raw, unrefined, extra-virgin oil from avocados, coconuts, flaxseeds, hemp, mustard seeds, peanuts, and sesame seeds.

Rock salt (Himalayan salt): Compared to purified sea salt, rock salt has a natural mineral composition, which is what gives it its color. Sea salt can be sold with or without iodine. Since iodine gets removed during the purification process, it must be added back in. If you cannot find rock/Himalayan salt, get sea salt but look for one with added iodine. Feel free to eat your meals without any added salt. We are very used to adding salt to our food, but it is not an essential component. Salt is naturally found in most vegetables and fruits.

Seeds: Chia, flax, hemp, pumpkin, and sesame seeds and pine nuts. These can be purchased raw or in powder form and added to smoothies or sprinkled over salads. Without adding any extra oil and salt, you can also roast these seeds in your own toaster oven between 325°F and 350°F till you can smell a nutty flavor emanating from the seeds. Be sure to use a Pyrex glass platter for roasting and not an aluminum or Teflon coated (non-stick) pan.

Spices, fresh and dried herbs: Basil, bay leaves, black pepper, cilantro, chives, culantro, cumin seeds, curry leaves, ginger, mint, oregano, rosemary, thyme, turmeric powder, and more.

Note that none of the above food items are processed, meaning they are as close to their natural state as possible. They are the basic ingredients for preparing a successful, nourishing, and healthy meal whenever you are ready to eat.

Shopping for Perishable Items

Do your own research to find out what is available in season in your locality. A general guide to seasonal foods is provided by the U.S.

Department of Agriculture.[62] Remember the importance of minimizing refrigeration in decisions about the locality of your produce and frequency of your shopping trips.

Fruits

Look for fresh, locally grown, organic fruit. The list is long, but you can focus on what grows in your region. Buying *fresh* fruit is important. When fresh, the fruits have tight skin and no (or hardly any) blemishes. When pressed gently with the fingertips, the fresh fruits have a slight give but they are not squishy. Look for fruits with unbroken skin and no dents, bruises, cuts, bug holes, or dark spots. When old, some fruits—for example strawberries and raspberries—begin to show mold growth. These are to be avoided. Smell the fruits. They should have a slight fruity smell indicating that they are ready to eat. Occasionally, you might get fresh fruits that are not ready to eat. These fruits can be left on the counter for a couple of days (or more) until they become ready to eat. Frozen fruits and fruits cut up and sold in plastic containers are to be avoided as much as possible because their freshness is uncertain.

Apples	Jackfruits	Passion fruits
Apricots	Jambuls	Papayas
Bananas and plantains	Kiwis	Peaches
Blackberries	Lychees	Pears
Blueberries	Mámon chino	Persimmons
Cherries	(Rambutan)	Prunes
Custard apples	Mangos	Plums
Chikoos	Melons	Pineapples
Coconuts	Nectarines	Pomegranates
Cranberries	Oranges	Raspberries
Figs	(blood oranges,	Strawberries
Grapefruits	clementines,	Soursops
Grapes	mandarins,	Watermelons
Guavas	tangerines)	

Vegetables

Look for fresh, locally grown, organic vegetables. The leaves should not be dried-up or wilted. Fresh vegetables have a particular sparkle that comes from moisture and cellular turgidity. Old vegetables lose moisture and cellular turgidity so they begin to look wilted. Make sure there are not cuts, bruises, or mold growth on the surface. Lettuce should not have brown, wet, or slimy leaves, which indicate that they have begun to rot. The list below is long, but you can focus on the vegetables that grow in your region.

Artichokes

Asparagus

Avocados

Broccoli

Beets and beet
    greens

Bitter melons

Butternut squash

Brussels sprouts

Cabbage

Carrots

Cauliflower

Celery

Celeriac
    (celery root)

Chayote

Cucumbers

Corn

Collard greens

Daikons

Eggplants

Endive

Fennel

Ginger

Garlic

Green peas

Green beans

Jerusalem artichoke

Jicama

Kohlrabi

Kale

Lettuce (especially
    arugula, and other
    dark-colored leaf
    varieties)

Mushrooms

Okra

Onions (including
    chives, leeks,
    shallots, and
    scallions)

Peppers

Pejiballe

Pumpkins

Purple cabbage

Radishes

Rhubarb

String beans

Spinach

Spaghetti squash

Summer squash

Sweet potatoes

Sweet peppers
    (chile dulce)

Tomatoes

Turnips

Watercress

Water chestnuts

Yams

Yucca

Zucchini

Meat, Eggs, and Seafood

If you plan on eating vegetarian foods while you're on the Ayurvedic reset diet, you need not buy these foods. However, if you do want to eat them, then buy them organic, as fresh as you can, and as close to the day you plan on eating them as possible, so you do not have to refrigerate them for long or freeze them at all. A note of caution: The spoilage rate is very high for meats, chicken, seafood, fish, and eggs if they are not refrigerated right away. You will be eating these foods mainly for their protein content, and protein does not deteriorate in the fridge/freezer. Even when frozen or refrigerated, meats must not be eaten past their expiration date and care should be taken to defrost them in the refrigerator so that germs do not begin to multiply at room temperature and cause food poisoning.

A note about buying already-frozen or processed meats and seafood: It is a practice to add cryoprotectants, like sodium phosphate, to raw, frozen chicken and other meats and seafood.[63] While these chemicals help meat products stay fresh in the freezer and not get freezer burn, they are toxic at higher concentrations and are only added to extend the shelf-life. Processed meats are filled with extenders during the manufacturing process.[64] Though they are ready to cook (e.g., hamburgers) and also can be ready to eat (e.g., corned beef), it would be best for you to stay away from them during your Ayurvedic reset diet.

ACTION 4: CLEANSE YOURSELF, INSIDE AND OUT

If you have followed the three actions I have outlined above, you have successfully put to rest (at least for now) any doubts and excuses you have concerning the Ayurvedic reset diet; cleaned the older, mainstream foods out of your fridge, freezer, and pantry; and refined your shopping habits to include healthy organic and seasonal foods where possible. It is now time to begin a cleansing process that focuses on you.

Cleansing the inner and outer body reinvigorates you and fosters a state of mind that is more receptive to positive influences. This will allow you to focus on the healing aspects of the Ayurvedic reset diet that you are about to start.

As we have learned, because of industrialization of the food supply chain, the eating habits of our species have become quite distorted in general. We routinely consume high amounts of sugars, refined flours, processed foods, and caffeine even without realizing that there is any need to change our habits. From this perspective, diving straight and deep into the Ayurvedic reset diet might pose a challenge to some individuals, mainly in the form of withdrawal symptoms. Some folks missing out on their daily dose of sugar begin to show signs and symptoms of withdrawal—for example depression, anxiety, changes in sleep pattern, cognitive issues, craving, lightheadedness, tingling, intense hunger, nausea, and fatigue.[65] Going cold turkey on all added sugars can bring up any or all of these symptoms and there would be a very strong desire to consume sugar again. The advantage of going cold turkey is that the withdrawal symptoms do not drag on and end sooner than later because the body begins to adapt quickly to the new reality of the sugarless eating habit. Some people prefer to drop sugar from their diet rather slowly. They do not experience intense withdrawal symptoms, because their body adapts gradually to the new reality of reduced sugar in their diet.

See pages 106–7 for information about caffeine withdrawal, another issue you may want to tackle *before* diving into the full diet.

As a daily habit, get up at dawn, preferably before the sun is up. This will immediately align you with the constructive, creative, tranquil forces of nature that operate at dawn. Before you start your day, brush your teeth and scrape your tongue and then drink eight ounces of warm water, plain or with one teaspoon of honey.

Next, take a shower. If you feel an urge to move your bowels, then attend to this urge first. If you do not feel the urge for a bowel movement right away, it will come a little later. Afterward, be sure to wash your lower body with soap and warm water again.

After your shower, wipe your eyes and nostrils and remove the crusts that formed overnight, comb or brush your hair, then dress in fresh, clean, comfortable clothes.

Please note that the Western and European habit of eating breakfast and having tea or coffee as soon as one gets up, even before brushing one's teeth or having a bowel movement, is not recommended in Ayurveda. This is because even though you brush and floss your teeth and use mouthwash before bedtime, enough bacteria build up in your mouth overnight to produce a slimy white or pale-yellow film that coats your teeth and tongue and creates a stale, offensive smell in your mouth. When you eat right after waking up, without brushing your teeth, you are allowing all those foul germs to get into your stomach. While these germs will not cause you any stomach upset, it is worth your trouble to ensure that you don't eat breakfast before cleaning, brushing, and thoroughly rinsing your mouth and scraping your tongue, because when you do so, you will see that you are more hungry and that your food tastes better.

A note about bowel movements: While there are as many bowel movement schedules as one can imagine, by following this routine of daily personal hygiene, drinking enough water, getting plenty of fiber in your food, and engaging in physical activity throughout the day, it is very likely that you will experience a change in your bowel movement schedule and instead of sitting on the throne once every other day, once a week, or once in a great while, you might be called to sit every morning at the same time, like clockwork.

And speaking of physical activity . . . I hate to give you the bad news, but I must. Just because you are switching to a different style of eating by engaging in the Ayurvedic reset diet does not mean that you get to become a couch potato. On the two days when you are drinking water only and then water and herb teas alternating, you can still do light walking. Later in the program, when you are eating three meals and snacks of fruits or vegetables, you will have plenty of energy to do a wide range of physical activities and exercises—even strenuous ones like weight lifting, biking, and swimming. There is no need to cut back on any of these activities, but be aware of your own personal physical state and if you require rest, by all means get some.

Our hunter-gatherer ancestors were constantly on the move while they were . . . you guessed it . . . hunting and gathering! They knew and walked their land like it was their personal and private backyard.

They ate one meal a day when food was available and spent much of the day running after prey. Women and children walked several miles on their land in search of edible fruits, nuts, berries, and roots. They were not sitting around just because they were fasting or eating one meal a day. The notion that our body will fall apart if we miss a meal or two is rather a new one and undoubtedly an outcome of the modern culture that promotes three meals a day so that industrially manufactured food can be consumed in shockingly large amounts.

However, the modern-day human body is no different from that of our hunter-gatherer ancestors. What is different is the speed at which we move (and how often) and the lack of interaction between our body and our environment. In general, the average modern human does not do much climbing, running, brisk walking, or swimming, or sit on the floor cross-legged, because these activities are not essential to his survival anymore. Our hunter-gatherer ancestors could not live without these basic skills.

In our own search for organic seasonal and local foods, the most physical activity we are going to get is walking around the farmers market or health food store. So how will we get enough exercise in our lives unless we intentionally make room for it?

As it turns out, sustained, continuous movement (like brisk walking) is good for the muscles, bones, joints, circulation, and even our mood. In a modern lifestyle, brisk walking, jogging, running, swimming, weight lifting, yoga, bicycling, skiing, and so on can be easily incorporated. We just have to get disciplined about doing the exercises of our choice on a daily basis. Consistency and routine help us overcome the voices in our mind that divert us from our purpose and make us lazy at times.

In my practice, several of my clients are committed to a simple exercise regimen that I frequently recommend called the Five Tibetans.[66]

It is easy to do and not extremely strenuous, and in about twenty minutes of basic yoga stretches that you can do in the comfort of your own home, every muscle and joint of your body gets a thorough workout. At the end of the set, you have slightly elevated heart and breathing rates, indicating that you have engaged in a moderately strenuous exercise.

However, it must be noted that no one exercise will work for everyone. Exercises can be tailor-made to suit one's age, physical condition, and mobility level. Take, for example, people over the age of fifty. As they enter the fifth decade of their life, it becomes more apparent that the activities they once enjoyed and engaged in with ease and comfort are becoming harder to do. It becomes easier to gain weight and harder to gain muscle mass. But the fact is that an exercise program can be designed to suit every decade of life. If you lead a sedentary life or have chronic health conditions, consult your health care provider before starting a new exercise program. Follow a safe program that suits your age and make sure to maintain good posture when you do it so that you can avoid injuries. Tom Buford, associate professor of medicine at the University of Alabama at Birmingham (UAB) and associate director of the UAB Center for Exercise Medicine, says that exercise programs suitable for your age, when done with care and proper form, can help you to stay fit and prevent injuries.[67]

One outdoor activity that provides a gentler form of exercise and is gaining momentum is forest bathing. All one has to do is go to the nearest available stretch of woods or park and walk about. People living in the cities and suburbs have little exposure, if any, to soil, uneven ground, plants, trees, greenery, or fresh air. A brief time spent forest bathing provides us with all these exquisite gifts of nature. Walking on uneven ground amid trees, birds, rustling leaves, moss, ferns, and even fungi, with little animals scurrying about, sunshine coming through the canopy, and a breeze wafting about revives our five senses, elevates our mood, and gives us clarity, focus, and a fresh perspective on our lives and our problems while our minds become still—as if they had been engaged in a deep meditation. Think about it, our hunter-gatherer ancestors did forest bathing *every day*! We can plan to do it at least twice a week.

Life is movement, and life is also stillness that can be experienced in moments of deep concentration and meditation. We need both for optimum health and well-being.

ACTION 5: SET THE "STAGE"

Today's eating style is to consume food while you are working, watching TV, talking loudly, fighting with someone, reading your email, texting, talking on the phone, walking on a busy street, or listening to music on your earphones. And often you are using knives, forks, spoons, and napkins. All of these distractions and interventions dissociate and disconnect you from your experience of eating food. You are not seeing, touching, smelling, tasting, and hearing food; you are busy doing something else while food is entering your mouth mechanically, robotically. In the modern method of eating, food is just a commodity for mindless consumption. It is not a source of nurturing for the body. If you lose touch with the spirit of the food, how can you expect this food to nourish your own spirit?

Luckily, you can successfully keep these modern-day diversions out of your dining area. After all, you have a remote for your TV, and you know how to turn off your devices and screens. Start with turning off the TV and cell phone. If you still have a landline, turn off the ringer and let the answering machine or service take the calls. Take off the earphones that feed music to your ears. When these devices are turned off, you will soon begin to notice that the earth is still spinning on her axis and has not come to a standstill just because you are offline/disconnected.

Put away newspapers, magazines, and even your work-related readings. Feed your pets before you sit down to eat so that they are not around the table soliciting food scraps, and make sure that any machines and gadgets that are meant to make household chores lighter—

dishwasher, washer-dryer, oven, etc.—are not beeping and ringing bells for your attention while you are sitting down to eat.

If you have company or family eating with you, keep the meal-time conversation to neutral topics and do not discuss politics, finances, world affairs, natural calamities, or your own emotional problems during your meal. Mealtime is sacred because that is when you are providing nutrition to all the koshas of your body, and maintaining an emotionally pleasant or at least neutral environment is essential.

Set aside a specific time when you will sit down to eat. Do not eat standing up or moving around. Make sure the eating area is well lit, nicely ventilated, and the right temperature for your needs. A clean, aesthetically pleasing dining area helps you enjoy your food more. You can light a candle and arrange fresh flowers on the table as a centerpiece and even have soft music playing in the background. The household and particularly the kitchen/dining area should be free from clutter, heaps of unfinished tasks, and reminders of your earlier meals. Neat and tidy surroundings help you focus on your meal with undivided attention.

It is a must that you wash your hands with soap and water before eating. Also, drink a glass of warm water half an hour before your meal. It helps clean out your mouth and flush your palate and taste buds so that your food will taste better. It also cleans the stomach by flushing out the old remnants of earlier meals, and signals it to get ready for the upcoming meal by starting to produce gastric juices.

If you are religious, you may say your prayer before the meal and offer the food to your god. If you are not religious, just eating food quietly without distractions and with an intention to heal yourself is a good idea.

What to Do If a Guest Arrives Unexpectedly

In my Indian culture, an unexpected mealtime guest is considered divine and welcomed with this expression from the Sanskrit language:

अतिथि देवो भव

Atithi Devo Bhava
The guest is equivalent to God

The unexpected mealtime guest is welcomed warmly and is offered the same food we happen to be eating. This is what I saw my parents do in my childhood home in India. There is no harm in practicing this old-world hospitality and warmth irrespective of where you live and what culture you belong to. "Do unto others as you would have them to do unto you," a Biblical saying, is enough of a motivation for anyone who finds an unexpected mealtime guest knocking on the door. You welcome them and treat them with generosity, as perchance, if you ever end up at someone's door at mealtime, you can hope to be treated well and received with warmth. What goes around indeed comes around.

When people are made to feel welcome, they feel happier and accepted, and this is a universal experience of people across all cultures. You can offer your guest a seat and give them a portion of the same food that you are eating. However, it is good to be respectful of the guest's eating styles. For example, if a vegetarian friend shows up unexpectedly during your mealtime, it might be disrespectful to offer her meat even if you're eating it. Instead you could offer her any of the other foods you are eating that fit into her own eating style.

DEALING WITH NOSY COLLEAGUES IN THE WORKPLACE

A workplace can be full of nice folks. It can also be teaming with pesky, nosy ones. However, if you want to keep your job, you will have to master the ability to navigate the dynamics and hierarchy that develop between coworkers due to their individual differences.

At work, if you get asked questions about your new Ayurvedic reset diet eating style, it is best to tell them in a straightforward manner about what you are doing and why. When friends and colleagues know what you are doing for your wellness, they generally become quite supportive of your efforts. Some of them might even express a wish to join you. On the other hand, they might offer contrasting ideas and try to get you off the program. In that case, you just exercise your willpower and ask them not to interfere. Tell them firmly that you're determined to stick with the Ayurvedic reset diet and ask them to mind their own beeswax and stop distracting you and trying to derail your plan. They will get the message because your determination and intention will come through loud and clear.

ACTION 6: SATISFY THE SENSES BY EATING WITH YOUR HANDS

Going back to the basics of cultivating a loving soulful relationship with food is possible when you learn the Ayurvedic method of engaging your five senses by eating food with your hands. Eating food is not a mechanical activity; it's a *sensory* one. While you eat, you can observe how you smell, see, touch, taste, and even hear food.

When I was a child, my parents taught me to eat with my fingers, and food was served on banana leaves. No plates, bowls, napkins, spoons, forks, knives, or dessert spoons were necessary. You do not have to go as far as serving food on banana leaves, but you can easily learn how to eat with your hands and begin to derive complete sensory satisfaction from the action of eating your food.

The Ayurvedic technique for eating with your hands follows a few simple guidelines:

- Keep your fingernails clipped very short and clean them daily.
- Wash your hands with soap and water before preparing meals.
- Go to the bathroom, if necessary, before sitting down to eat so that your meal is not interrupted. Be sure to wash your hands and

nails with soap and water and dry them well with a clean towel afterward.

- Arrange all of the foods that you are going to eat so that they are within easy reach on your table. If you are at home, you can also sit down cross-legged on a simple cushion or floor mat. Traditionally when people sit on the floor to eat, the food to be served is arranged on the floor too, and a table is not necessary.
- Have a glass of water available, but note that you do not have to take a sip after every bite of food. Drinking water when you're eating is thought to dilute gastric juices and gives you an inaccurate sense of fullness. As a result, you end up eating less and soon after mealtime you feel hungry and go looking for snacks.
- Serve yourself a small quantity of food.
- Keep your left hand free and clean for helping yourself to additional servings.
- Before you start eating, take a moment or two to observe and enjoy the texture, appearance, color, and smell of your food.
- With your right hand, using all five fingers, pick up a small quantity of food from your plate.
- As you place the food in your mouth, enjoy the flavor, aroma, and texture of your food. Pay attention to the crunching sounds that come from chewing. With your mouth closed, chew the food long enough to turn it into the texture of a soft porridge. Then swallow.

BENEFITS OF EATING FOOD WITH ALL FIVE FINGERS

Touching food with all five fingers allows all the nerve endings on your fingertips to be influenced by the food. Using your fingertips also encourages you to take only a small amount of food at a time so that it does not spill out of your grip, and since you're not completely filling your mouth each time you take a bite, there is enough room to move the food around and allow it to mix with the saliva as you're chewing it. This extended chewing process excites the salivary glands to produce enough saliva for the job and helps the roughage in the food to clean your teeth while you are eating.

When you touch, see, smell, taste and hear your food, all five sensory organs of your body become active, and they carry the sensory information to your brain. The brain actually understands that you are in the process of eating and enjoying your food, and this sensory satisfaction is necessary for the stomach to produce the satiety signal that tells you to stop eating as soon as you are full. There is no need to overeat because all five of your senses are satisfied.

6

The Ayurvedic Reset Diet

Eight-, Six-, and One-Week Protocols

If you have completed all the preparations listed in chapter 5, you are fully equipped to begin the actual process of the Ayurvedic reset diet and have proven that you have enough resolve to successfully complete it. And I want to assure you that while you may be eating fewer *types* of food at first, you will still have plenty to eat.

Important note: If you have any serious medical condition, please consult with your doctor before making changes to your diet. Pregnant and nursing women, young children, and those recovering from surgery should not engage the Ayurvedic reset diet. Pregnant and nursing women must have access to as much food as they need, when they need it. They can always choose healthier options, but they must make sure that they are getting enough food and all the necessary nutrients. Likewise, restricting food or limiting the availability is not in the best interest of young children who are still experiencing so much mental and physical development. In addition, when young children hit a growth spurt, they want to eat a lot and should do so. Post-surgery the body is recovering from anesthesia as well as the surgical procedure and is in a compromised state. Foods must be introduced gradually and sudden changes in quality and quantity of food must be avoided.

KEEPING A JOURNAL

Before you begin your first week of the diet, buy a journal or notebook in which you can plan out your week and keep track of what you eat. You will also want to make note of any emotions and feelings that are associated with your food intake and what thoughts come up repeatedly. What cravings and aversions come up for you? How does your food taste? While keeping this journal, you will make each meal into a session for mindfulness.

At the end of Weeks 1, 2, 3, and 4, be sure to weigh yourself and write down your weight in the journal. Also, note the level of your daily energy and your ability to focus. Do not be upset if significant weight loss has not happened. You will be consuming plenty of water and plenty of vegetables or fruits as well. Although you will be cutting your calorie intake, your body will be getting plenty of food and will not go into starvation mode.

At the conclusion of your Ayurvedic reset diet, spend some time looking through this journal to see how your relationship to your food, your bodily symptoms, your emotions, and your overall disposition changed as you progressed and went deeper into the Ayurvedic reset diet.

EIGHT-, SIX-, AND ONE-WEEK PROTOCOLS

The full Ayurvedic reset diet is to be undertaken for a short period only, no longer than eight weeks at a time. The first four weeks consist of fasting on water or water and herbal tea for the first two days of each week (step 1) and then eating two weeks of vegetables only and then two weeks of fruits only (step 2). Then the plan proceeds to a total of four more weeks in which you will mix/combine foods from various food groups (step 3) by eating from one food group only at each meal. Within this time period, your gut will cleanse, detox, and repair itself, and the other healing processes of the body will kick in.

It is also possible to undertake a six- or one-week protocol, and instructions for doing so are provided later in the chapter.

THE EIGHT-WEEK PROTOCOL

The following sections provide instructions for the full eight-week Ayurvedic reset diet protocol.

WEEKS 1 AND 2: VEGETABLES ONLY

WEEK 1, DAY 1
FASTING ON ROOM TEMPERATURE OR WARM WATER ONLY

The first two days of the Ayurvedic reset diet are fasting days. This means that you are not going to eat any solids or drink any other liquid but water. However, you can drink as much water as you need and can possibly drink. You will be peeing a lot but that is okay. *A note to diabetics: Studies are coming up that support the idea that type 2 diabetics could fast safely if they can keep an eye on their hypoglycemia event.*[68]

Drink at least one eight-ounce glass of water every hour. You can have it warm or at room temperature. Avoid drinking ice cold water with ice floating in it. If you want, you can squeeze a slice of lemon into the water, but do not add sugar, salt, honey, or anything else.

As you begin to drink water, slow down a bit. There is no rush. Hold the water in your mouth for a little while. Savor its taste. Move it around. Let it get mixed with saliva. After all, water is the most important ingredient of your food and also your body. It keeps you alive just like air does. Why be in a hurry? Drink your water slowly, mindfully, as if it is divine nectar.

It is better to avoid chlorinated water and carbonated (bubbly) water. If you have access to water from your own well that is best. If not, you can drink filtered tap water. If you must buy bottled water, then look for it in glass bottles. If these are not available, then look for plastic bottles that do not contain Bisphenol A (BPA). This chemical leaches from plastic bottles into water and gets into your bloodstream. BPA is known to mimic the action of estrogen in the body.

Possible Effects of Detoxing Your Body

While fasting on water only, you might experience some lethargy, exhaustion, hunger, need for rest, and maybe light-headedness as well. When you need rest, take rest. If you feel hungry, go for your cup of water. While feeling lethargic, take a short walk and get some fresh air. While these sensations might be new for you, these are not problematic. You can ride them out and continue fasting, because these are simple signs that your body is getting rid of unwanted old junk from your digestive tract and elsewhere.

WEEK 1, DAY 2
FASTING ON WATER ALTERNATING WITH HERBAL TEAS

Day 2 of fasting is very important because it extends the cleansing and regeneration time given to the tissues and organs of the digestive tract and your excretory system. When the gastrointestinal and excretory system is not constantly dealing with incoming foods and metabolites, it is not only getting cleaned but is also repairing its cells and tissues.

You may not have a bowel movement on this day as you did not eat anything the day before. But if you did not have a bowel movement before starting your Day 1 of water intake, your bowels might want to clear themselves out. Honey and plenty of water provide the energy and pressure necessary to create a bowel movement.

Herbal teas are steeped in boiling hot water for three to five minutes and then consumed. You can add a squeeze of lemon and a teaspoon of honey if you like. Drink a cup of herbal tea alternating with a glass of plain water—again, one drink every hour. Or you might prefer to just extend the water-only fast to Day 2 and not bother with herbal teas. That is quite fine too. However, herbal teas with some honey added provide a slight amount of energy, satisfy the need for warm drinks, increase the metabolism in the body, and break the monotony of drinking just water for two days in a row.

Local, Raw, Organic Honey and Type 2 Diabetes

There are studies that support the view that even people with type 2 diabetes can eat local, raw, and organic honey, and if they do so, they might even experience a reduction in body weight and blood lipids as well as glucose.[69]

Several different types of herbal tea are available. Choose teas made from organic herbs. Anise, basil, black pepper, cardamom, chamomile, clove, cinnamon, coriander, cumin, turmeric, dandelion, fennel, ginger, green tea, hibiscus, lemon balm, licorice, mint, rooibos, spearmint, and senna are some of the teas that can help with cleansing the digestive system and its glands as well as help the kidneys with diuretic action.[70] A word of caution about cinnamon tea: cinnamon is known in Ayurveda to bring down blood pressure as well as blood sugar. So use this particular tea with care if your blood pressure and sugar are not being controlled.

Caffeine Withdrawal

During these two fasting days, you will come to know if you are addicted to caffeine by whether or not you experience withdrawal symptoms such as headache, fatigue, anxiety, irritability, low energy, depressed mood, listlessness, jitteriness, and lethargy.[71]

If you experience these symptoms, caffeine intake must have become a habit and breaking it in one day can be problematic. As you begin your water-only fast, make sure your caffeine supply is available, at least the first cup of tea or coffee that you drink in the morning. With your dose of caffeine nearby, you can put off taking it as long as withdrawal symptoms do not come up. However, when you feel the first stirrings of these symptoms, have a glass of warm water first, then drink your cup of tea or coffee, then have another glass of warm water afterward. Drinking strong tea and coffee on an empty stomach can produce a burning sensation as well as an increased acidity in the stomach. Diluting these beverages with warm water before and after drinking them can help reduce these effects.

Each subsequent day, try consuming a little less of your caffeinated beverage. Hopefully within a few days you will be able to omit it completely. If you continue to experience withdrawal symptoms, then you have to make a concession and allow yourself to have your caffeine; however, make it as diluted as possible. On nonfasting days, avoid drinking these beverages on an empty stomach, as they are known to increase acidity. Eat your vegetable or fruit meal and then have your coffee or tea in a very diluted form.

This intake of one cup of caffeinated tea or coffee is *only* to reduce the effects of withdrawal. Avoid adding sugar or cream, and avoid decaffeinated coffee or decaffeinated tea while on the diet. (Note that herbal tea is naturally caffeine free, this is different than the decaffeination of naturally caffeinated substances, which usually requires a process using chemicals that are harmful and leaves residual caffeine.)

Fruit Juices

Fruit juices—the store-bought ones, even if they are organic—contain the color, taste, and sugar content of the fruit, but because the pulp is filtered out and removed, they are missing the fiber, minerals, and vitamins you would get from eating the fruit itself. You basically end up getting a large amount of sugar and nothing else.

More importantly here, however, is that the very purpose of fasting is to abstain from eating all other food groups/nutrients and allow *zero-calorie* water the maximum chance to clean your digestive and excretory system, and since fruit juices are full of calories from sugar, they are in the "don't even think about it" list during water-only fasting days.

Alcoholic Beverages

While fasting on water only, and then water alternating with herbal teas, your stomach is going to be completely empty. Alcoholic beverages are sources of empty calories, and drinking them on an empty stomach means that they will move to the small intestine for digestion very quickly.[72] All the effects of alcohol get quite magnified because of this, and the liver now has to metabolize the alcohol when it is supposed to be resting. Drinking alcohol during fasting, and, further along the line, during the mono-diet stage of the Ayurvedic reset diet is again on the "don't even think about it" list.

Enemas

The purpose of fasting is to cleanse the inner body. If, during the two days of water only and water plus herbal teas, you have had no urge to move your bowels, an enema will be required.[73]

Enemas should be taken, if necessary, before you start eating again, which is scheduled from Day 3 onward. *Please note that people who have injuries or have had recent surgery should not try the enema treatment at home.* Before any new food goes into your system, the old, leftover feces must be eliminated. For this purpose, purchase an enema bag from a pharmacy. The best time to take an enema is early morning, before starting the other activities of your day. Read the instructions below as well as on the enema bag package. You'll want to be as close to a toilet as possible. Lubricate the nozzle and fill up the enema bag with lukewarm water. Lie down on your left side in a comfortable position. Insert the nozzle up your anus and allow the warm water to enter your body. Once the full contents of the enema bag are internalized, remain in the comfortable position on your left side. Let the warm water irrigate the rectum and colon. Within the next few minutes, you will feel a very strong urge to evacuate your bowels. Stool will come out with explosive force, and the bowel will continue to evacuate for a while. Sit patiently on the throne and complete the evacuation. Then wash yourself very well with soap and water and take a shower as well for better hygiene.

Further along the Ayurvedic reset diet, you can use an enema if you have not had any bowel movement in a day. Normally, you will make at least one bowel movement daily if not two, simply because the meals are designed with very high fiber content.

WEEK 1, DAYS 3, 4, 5, 6, AND 7
MONO-DIET ON VEGETABLES ONLY

These five days of Week 1 are fundamental to the Ayurvedic reset diet because this is when you are going to practice a mono-diet, where you focus on eating one type of food at a time. These days are devoted to eating vegetables only for breakfast, lunch, dinner, and snacks. No other foods are allowed. *A note to diabetics: Be sure to avoid vegetables that have high glycemic index and are full of simple starches; for example, beet root, potatoes, sweet potatoes, corn, carrots, tomatoes, yellow squashes, pumpkins, etc.*

Although you are only eating vegetables, you can eat as much of them as you need. You are not depriving yourself or starving. As a result, you will not be extremely hungry and thus you will have a better chance of staying on the plan and bringing it to a successful conclusion.

Many diets fail because they offer too little in terms of eating experience and are designed to help you lose weight drastically. The Ayurvedic reset diet has a different agenda. It is designed to help you clean the gut without experiencing starvation. You can get up to 700 or 800 calories from just one type of food and that is sufficient, for a short duration, for cleaning up your system. In chapter 5, I gave you a step-by-step method for eating food with your hands to satisfy all five of your senses, so you will not be inclined to overeat as if you were not going to see any more food the next day (see pages 99–101).

The best guide for knowing how much to eat is your own hunger.

Eat enough vegetables to fill your stomach. You do not have to starve yourself while you are practicing the Ayurvedic reset diet, and there is no need to overeat at any given meal either, because you can always have a vegetable snack between meals.

Eat Just One Type of Vegetable for Each Meal (or Each Day)

In therapeutic applications of the Ayurvedic reset diet, people have obtained brilliant results by eating just one type of vegetable for over two weeks, for all meals and snacks.[74] For the best curative outcomes, it is best to stick with this recommendation. However, for the general purposes of cleansing, regeneration, rejuvenation, and weight loss, it is okay to eat different vegetables each day, but not in the same meal (and not cooked together). So, on Week 1 of vegetables only, you would eat only one type of vegetable—broccoli, for example—for breakfast, then either continue with just broccoli throughout the day or choose another type for each meal, say, carrots for lunch and sweet potatoes (with skin) for dinner. This allows the digestive system to fully extract all the nutrients from that one type of vegetable and then focus its attention on extracting nutrients from reserved fats and unwanted tissues in the body before the next meal.

For example, combining potatoes and sweet potatoes, which are mainly carbohydrates, with celery or cucumber or lettuce, which are mainly fibers, creates an overload of carbohydrates and insoluble fibers. This combination might give you a lot of bloating, distension, and flatulence from accumulated gases.

Choosing Vegetables

Select the vegetables that you enjoy or pick some from the list on page 90. These vegetables should be seasonal and available locally when you are beginning your Ayurvedic reset diet. Since most vegetables have to be refrigerated, and refrigeration kills some vitamins, it is best to buy small quantities, especially if you can shop twice or more every week.

This might be a good time to try some new vegetables that you have not eaten before.

Cooking Vegetables

You can eat vegetables raw, slightly sautéed in olive or coconut oil, or steamed, with or without salt. Avoid deep-frying, grilling, and overcooking because these processes not only kill nutrients but also cause the formation of carcinogenic compounds in the vegetables. For example, potatoes and sweet potatoes, boiled in the skin and eaten with skin, are good for you. (However, please note that due to carbohydrate overload from potatoes and sweet potatoes, even if they are eaten with skin, you may not have an urge for a bowel movement. It is recommended therefore that when you eat these vegetables, you consider taking an enema if you do not have a bowel movement per your daily routine.) However, when the potatoes are peeled and deep fried in oil that has been used and reused many times over, they lose their vitamins and become poisonous to the body because of the trans fatty acids imparted to them from the overused oil. When starches and proteins are cooked at very high temperatures and browned/burned, they undergo glycation, a process that leads to the formation of carcinogens.[75] The same goes for grilled vegetables that become dark brown or black in the process of grilling.

Vegetable Recipes

This section includes a few simple methods for cooking vegetables during the Ayurvedic reset diet.

Stir-Fried Vegetables

The vegetables that do not have to be cooked thoroughly can be stir fried. These include red and yellow onions, spinach, kale, radishes, garlic, carrots, peas, celery, horseradish, green beans, ginger, white cabbage, purple cabbage, cauliflower, broccoli, chayote, tomatoes, and peppers.

Remember that at this stage of the diet, you should be stir-frying just one type of vegetable per meal or day. Wash the vegetable and peel it if necessary. Then chop it into small bite-sized pieces. For two cups of vegetables, use one teaspoon of coconut oil or olive oil. Heat the oil gently, add the chopped vegetables, then turn the heat to high and stir fry for five minutes. Add salt and pepper and a squeeze of lemon to taste.

Steamed Vegetables

Chayote, cauliflower, carrots, broccoli, squash (including pumpkins), sweet potatoes, and potatoes taste better when they are steamed till a fork can be inserted without resistance. Once the vegetable is well steamed, it can be pureed with water and turned into a thick soup, or it can be mashed with a fork, seasoned to taste, and eaten like mashed potatoes. Here's a recipe that works like a charm: Chop 2 cups of your vegetable of choice and steam it until it becomes quite soft, and you can run a fork through it. Add ⅓ cup of coconut water and puree the steamed vegetable mix in a blender. Add salt and pepper to taste and a small dab of coconut oil for extra flavor.

Vegetable Soup

Using just one vegetable you can make a batch of soup that provides enough for a day of meals. Chop 5 or 6 cups of your chosen vegetable. Bring ten cups of water to a boil. Add the chopped vegetables, then turn down the heat and allow them to simmer until they become tender. Add the juice of a full lemon, salt and pepper to taste, and a full cup of chopped cilantro.

Raw Vegetables

For those vegetables that can be eaten raw, make a dressing with one-part olive oil, one-part vinegar or lemon juice, one tablespoon chopped garlic, and salt and pepper to taste.

Remember to Drink Water

During the vegetable-only week, you still need to drink lots of water. A good calculation for how much water you need is to weigh yourself, divide the weight by half, then convert that amount into ounces.[76] For example: If your body weight is 140 pounds, half of that is 70 pounds. That means, your daily fluid intake from water and teas should be 70 ounces, or about nine 8-ounce glasses. This is the amount of water (including herbal teas) that you will be drinking during vegetable-only week and throughout your reset diet.

Week 2, Day 1
Fasting on Room Temperature or Warm Water Only

Again, it is time to be fasting on water only and let to your digestive tract rest. As you did in Week 1, Day 1, drink a cup of water, either warm or at room temperature, every hour.

Week 2, Day 2
Fasting on Water Alternating with Herbal Teas

On the second day, you will again be fasting on water alternating with herbal teas. Drink a cup of tea alternating with a cup of plain water, one drink every hour.

Week 2, Days 3, 4, 5, 6, and 7
Ayurvedic Ieset Diet on Vegetables Only

You will again be practicing the mono-diet with vegetables only. Remember to stick with one type of vegetable per day for breakfast, lunch, dinner, and snacks (see below).

Snacks during Vegetables-Only Weeks

While you are eating only vegetables three times a day, you are going to be quite hungry for some snacks. Have a supply of a vegetable that you are eating that day cut up in raw form (if it can be eaten in raw form) available for you to snack on. This snack can be the size of a small meal so you do not feel too hungry. Some vegetables—eggplant, potatoes, sweet potatoes, and pejiballe, for example—cannot be eaten raw. They must be cooked well.

WEEKS 3 AND 4: FRUITS ONLY

WEEK 3, DAY 1
FASTING ON ROOM TEMPERATURE OR WARM WATER ONLY

As in Weeks 1 and 2, you will be fasting on water only. Drink a glass of room temperature or warm water only, once every hour.

WEEK 3, DAY 2
FASTING ON WATER ALTERNATING WITH HERBAL TEAS

You will again be fasting on water alternating with herbal teas. Drink warm or room temperature water alternating with herbal tea. Since in the weeks ahead you will be eating fruits only, you will be getting plenty of sweet taste, so you might prefer to avoid adding honey to your herbal tea. That is okay.

WEEK 3, DAYS 3, 4, 5, 6, AND 7
AYURVEDIC RESET DIET ON FRUITS ONLY

After doing Days 1 and 2 on water and water alternating with herbal teas, you will spend the next five days eating fruits only. In these two weeks, there are no vegetables to think about unless you are a diabetic. People who are diabetics can continue two more weeks of eating vegetables only as mentioned above. However, if they can manage their blood sugar within range, then they might be able to do the fruits-only step of the Ayurvedic reset diet as long as they choose whole fruits with a low glycemic index like berries.

Eat Just One Type of Fruit Each Meal (or Each Day)

As with vegetables, people have obtained wonderful therapeutic results by eating just one type of fruit for over two weeks, for all meals and snacks.[77] However, for the general purposes of cleansing, regeneration, rejuvenation, and weight loss, it is okay to eat one type of fruit—apples, for instance—for breakfast, then another type, say blueberries, for lunch, and so on. This allows the digestive system to fully extract all the nutrients from one type of fruit and then focus its attention on extracting nutrients from reserved fats and unwanted tissues in the body.

During your two weeks of vegetables only, your digestive system was trained to extract all the nutrients from one type of vegetable at a time. Now it will do the same with fruits. Please note that due to the high sugar content of fruits, you might experience a little bloating/gas, but since you are eating fruits only and not combining them with meat, etc., the bloating and gas will be minimal.

Choosing Fruits

Feel free to eat any fruit that is in season and available locally. See the list on page 89 for some ideas. Since you will be eating fruit for breakfast, lunch, dinner, and even snacks, make sure to get a good supply of the fruits you are planning to eat. But remember that the shelf life of fruit is relatively short, so you may need to shop for it more than once a week.

Homemade Fruit Juices

Please do not waste your time and money juicing fruit. When fruits are juiced, you end up throwing out all the fiber and skin, and therefore, all the complex carbohydrates get thrown out too, leaving you with just the watery part of the fruit, some color, and a bunch of simple sugars. When you drink fruit juices, you can get hungry very quickly, and your blood sugar can fluctuate too much, making you jittery when blood sugar is high and lethargic when blood sugar gets low.

However, making fruit smoothies with coconut water is a good idea because when you make a smoothie the entire fiber content of the fruit can be retained, as it is not filtered and thrown out.

❧ ❧ ❧

Fruit Smoothie

To make enough smoothie for a single meal, simply blend 2 cups of cut-up fruit and half a cup of coconut water at high speed until the entire fruit content is chopped up and blended with coconut water. Do not add any additional sugar.

WEEK 4, DAY 1
FASTING ON ROOM TEMPERATURE OR WARM WATER ONLY

You are back to fasting and drinking either room temperature or warm water only once every hour.

WEEK 4, DAY 2
FASTING ON WATER ALTERNATING WITH HERBAL TEAS

On the second day, as you have done before, alternate drinking warm or room temperature water with herbal teas with or without honey.

WEEK 4, DAYS 3, 4, 5, 6, AND 7
MONO-DIET ON FRUITS ONLY

As you did in Week 3, stay with fruits and fruit smoothies for breakfast, lunch, dinner, and snacks. *Remember to figure the amount of water to drink per day by dividing your body weight in half and converting that amount to ounces per day.*

SNACKS DURING FRUITS-ONLY WEEKS

Have a box of cut-up fruit and a bottle of fruit smoothie available so you can snack on them between mealtimes.

YOUR RESTED AND RENEWED DIGESTIVE SYSTEM

At this point in the Ayurvedic reset diet, your digestive system has learned to digest just one type of food, and your body has learned to live on a reduced calorie intake. Because of the high fiber content of fresh vegetables and fruits, your stool formation and elimination has become regularized. Old fecal deposits from habitual constipation have been flushed out during the two days per week of water intake. You have been through an internal cleanse, and you have allowed the GI tract to repair its lining, strengthen the digestive juices, and flush out old debris from the nooks and corners of the digestive tract. Because it didn't have to work overtime to digest heavy, rich foods, your digestive system was able to spend all its time digesting simple foods like vegetables and fruits, so it has had sufficient rest. You are now ready to start including other food groups in your meals.

WEEKS 5, 6, 7, AND 8: MIXING/COMBINING FOOD GROUPS BY EATING THEM AT DIFFERENT MEALS

After being on two weeks of vegetables only and two weeks of fruits only or, if you're a diabetic, a full four weeks of vegetables only, you are about to enter an exciting step of the Ayurvedic reset diet. During the last four weeks of the eight-week protocol, you will begin to add grain and protein sources back into your meals. However, since you are still on an isolation diet, you will be including them in a manner that allows the body to digest one food group completely before it is exposed to the next one. In this way you will be staying clear of viruddha ahara.

But remember that you need to remain fully aware of what, when, and how you eat and avoid indulging in the historical dietary errors where you freely mixed all the different food groups into one meal. The switch to including various food groups is going to be a deliberate, gentle, and gradual process, so it does not shock your body.

Step 3, the last step of the Ayurvedic reset diet, is the step when you confidently apply the body wisdom and the lessons that you have learned during steps 1 and 2 of the diet.

You can remain on this step for four weeks, but every week must be preceded by one day of fasting on water only and one day of fasting on water alternated with herbal tea. Such fasting will help the body to continue to repair itself, regenerate healthy tissues, and digest unwanted tissues. Two days of fasting per week will also help reduce your overall calorie intake so that you are better able to manage your weight and still enjoy a wide range of foods that you eat in moderation at different times.

WEEKS 5, 6, 7, AND 8, DAY 1
FASTING ON ROOM TEMPERATURE OR WARM WATER ONLY

As before, you will be fasting on water only, one cup every hour.

WEEKS 5, 6, 7, AND 8, DAY 2
FASTING ON WATER ALTERNATING WITH HERBAL TEAS

Again, just as before, you will alternate water and herbal tea with honey, one drink per hour.

WEEKS 5, 6, 7, AND 8, DAYS 3, 4, 5, 6, AND 7
MIXING/COMBINING FOOD GROUPS

Follow the isolation meal plan below for Days 3 through 7 for the next four weeks. Every day before you have your breakfast, brush your teeth, drink eight ounces of warm water, and do the rest of your morning routine as described in "Action 4: Cleanse Yourself, Inside and Out" on pages 91–96.

ISOLATION MEAL PLAN FOR
WEEKS 5 THROUGH 8

The following meal plan will allow you to eat from all the food groups every day while still isolating them to avoid viruddha ahara. Please note that although you are starting to include various food groups, you are still going to stay away from wheat, wheat flour, sugar, and dairy.

WATER INTAKE

The calculation for daily water intake throughout this meal plan remains the same as before—half of your body weight converted into ounces. As a general rule, drink water an hour after each meal and snack. Since you will be eating a variety of food groups now, you may not be that thirsty. But do stick to this water-intake rule. It will make you feel full, so you will not be overly hungry in between meals. It will also help with the routine cleansing of the body. With a large daily intake of water along with high-fiber foods, you will not have any concerns about constipation.

COOKING FOOD IN BULK

To save time and make meal preparation easier and more convenient, you may be tempted to cook food in bulk, refrigerate or even freeze it, and then reheat it for future meals. However, already-cooked foods have to be thawed if frozen and reheated if refrigerated, and the process of repeatedly thawing and reheating kills the nutritive quality and taste of foods. And according to Ayurveda, stale food does not have any life force, or prana, left in it, so if you're eating leftovers, you're missing out on that source of energy, too.

BREAKFAST: CARBOHYDRATE AND FAT INTAKE

Breakfast is the time to combine carbohydrates and healthy fats in the form of smoothies, nuts, seeds, and fruits to give you the necessary energy to get through the morning.

First prepare a smoothie by blending a whole fruit of your choice and coconut water. If coconut water does not agree with you, then just plain water will do. You can also add powdered seeds like hemp and flax into your smoothie to give it a thicker texture.

Along with the smoothie, eat ¼ cup of seeds and nuts such as pistachios, almonds, cashews, Brazil nuts, chestnuts, pecans, peanuts, walnuts, macadamias, hazelnuts, pine nuts, flaxseeds, sesame seeds, pumpkin seeds, and any other nuts and seeds that you enjoy. Buy small quantities of nuts and seeds, because the oils present in them can oxidize and become stale if these foods are not stored properly. Nuts and seeds should be stored in air-tight containers.

Nuts and seeds contain, on average, 10 percent protein, 15 percent carbohydrates, and 75 percent unsaturated fats. These fats create satiety, so after eating nuts you'll feel full for a long time. You can combine the nuts and seeds or eat one type one day and another type another day. You can eat them raw or toast them lightly.

⌇ ⌇ ⌇

Toasting Nuts and Seeds

When toasting, please make sure that the nuts and seeds do not burn or turn very brown in the process—because if they do, they will lose their nutritional quality and taste bitter. To toast, preheat a toaster oven to 325 to 350°F. Spread the nuts or seeds in a single layer in a Pyrex dish. Heat the seeds or nuts for twelve to fifteen minutes or until you smell a nutty aroma. Make sure to stir and turn the nuts or seeds after six minutes of roasting.

Almonds can be soaked overnight and eaten with the brown skin on the next morning. Overnight soaking makes them easier to chew and starts the germination process so that additional, highly nutritious enzymes become available to you as you eat these nuts.

Please note that candied nuts available in the market are not an option. Even when they are organic, they are processed and contain a lot of sugar.

You can also prepare and eat a bowl of cut-up fruit of your choice. You can eat one type of fruit alone or mix a few fruits together. Be sure to leave the skin on if it can be eaten. I have found that preparing a mixed-fruit bowl has one disadvantage: the portions of unused fruit must be refrigerated and that very quickly begins to bring down the texture and quality of the fruit. Therefore, my recommendation is to cut up just one type of fruit and eat it up in a day, so you won't have to store a large quantity of mixed fruit in the refrigerator.

Digestion Time for Fruits, Nuts, and Seeds

Smoothies and very watery fruits like watermelon will digest and exit the stomach in about twenty to thirty minutes. More dense fruits such as papaya, pineapple, and apple take about forty minutes. Nuts are slower to digest; they take about two to three hours.[78]

Even with a small midmorning snack around 10:00 a.m., your stomach will have plenty of time to digest and pass along the foods that you ate at breakfast.

SNACK

A small bowl of fruit would be sufficient for a midmorning snack, and the best time to eat it is around 10:00 a.m. or when you feel hungry again after your breakfast.

LUNCH

When you wake up at dawn and have your breakfast between 6:00 and 7:00 a.m., you will be ready for your midday meal by noon. At this meal, you are going to include foods with complex carbohydrates and fiber, namely grains and vegetables.

Cook whole grain quinoa and brown, black, or wild rice with bran, barley, and/or oats. Most of these grains come with a recipe on how to cook them, but you can reduce the cooking time by presoaking the grains using the following technique.

Cooking Grains

Measure out the amount of grain you are about to cook. Rinse and wash the grain with water then drain thoroughly. Now add the amount of water recommended for cooking and let the grain soak in it for an hour. Then begin cooking on low heat until all the water is absorbed. Cooked in this fashion, grains retain their texture but become soft and nice to eat without getting too mushy. Adding salt and oil while the grains are cooking is an option, but they are not necessary.

You can steam vegetables or cook them in stir-fries or soups. You can have corn on the cob, but avoid tortillas because they are made from refined corn flour. Add a large salad in this meal and include different vegetables that can be eaten raw. At this stage, when you are beginning to combine foods, you can start mixing various vegetables together as you cook them. Salads can also be a mix of lettuce leaves and cut-up raw vegetables.

Ratio of Vegetables to Grains

It would be tempting to load up on your favorite grain because you have been eating only vegetables and fruits for the past four weeks. But do remember that all grains are, in truth, seeds of various plants and are harder to digest and take much longer too. It would be wise to include them in small quantities.

As a general rule for your lunch, imagine four sections on your plate. Fill up two sections with raw vegetables and salads, one section with cooked vegetables, and the last remaining section with cooked grains (see page 123). Since grains are primarily a source of carbohydrates, you will be eating only a small quantity of them. In this way, your body will get enough carbohydrates to produce energy and heat, but not so many that they have to be stored away as glycogen and converted into fat.

Digestion Time for Grains and Vegetables

The time it takes for grains and vegetables to complete the gastric stage of digestion varies. Vegetables are digested in the stomach in around sixty minutes. Grains take about ninety minutes. In less than six hours, these foods will move out of the stomach and go into the small intestine for the next stage of digestion.

SNACK

After the midday meal of grains, vegetables, and salads, you may not need a snack. But if you do, then a handful of cut-up vegetables or nuts makes a very filling snack.

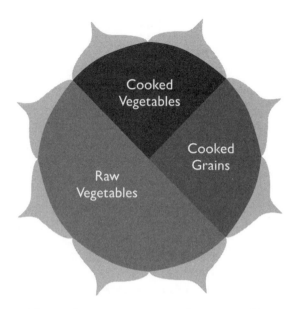

*Platter showing proportions of raw vegetables,
cooked vegetables, and grains*

DINNER

Dinner is the time to eat protein. Vegetarians will get their protein from plant-based sources, while meat eaters will stick mostly with protein from animals.

Vegetarians and Plant-Based
Sources of Protein

In this meal, vegetarians will get their protein from the vegetable kingdom, including French lentils, dals, black beans, sprouted mung beans, kidney beans, garbanzo beans, soybeans, etc. Nuts and seeds can be eaten again at this meal for texture and crunchiness, but fruits, vegetables, and grains should not be included.

Legumes contain protein, but they also contain almost double the amount of carbohydrates. However, these carbohydrates are complex and are made up of a mix of soluble and insoluble fiber, which makes them slow to digest. Eating legumes separate from grains, fruits, and vegetables ensures that the legumes do not languish in the digestive tract while the other foods are digested and absorbed into the body for further metabolism.

The cultures that practice vegetarian cuisine have an understanding of how legumes and grains complement each other. Legumes are low in the essential amino acid methionine but high in the amino acid lysine. Grains, on the other hand, are low in lysine but high in methionine. Mixing these two food groups, as in rice and dal (India), black beans and rice (Costa Rica), beans and corn tortillas (Mexico), tofu and rice (Asia), and peanut butter and bread (United States) is a common practice to ensure that the body receives a balanced supply of nutrients and amino acids.[79]

Although in the Ayurvedic reset diet you are going to eat legumes all by themselves and not combine them with grains, you will still get enough nutrition and all the essential amino acids because you are eating grains for lunch and legumes for dinner. The difference is that you are not mixing them in the same meal as you have been doing all your life.

Digestion Time for Protein from Legumes

Legumes take about three hours to move out of the gastric phase of digestion. However, by the time the partially digested legumes clear out of the stomach and reach the small intestine, the carbohydrates and fibers from your earlier meals of the day (breakfast of fruits and nuts, lunch of vegetables and grains) have already been digested and moved out of the small intestine. These carbohydrates and fibers are not trapped along with slow-digesting legumes, swelling up with water absorption and fermenting to make gas. Legumes get to have the entire small intestine area to themselves, so they can undergo a thorough digestion.

Meat Eaters and Protein from Animal Sources

At dinner, you can have beef, lamb, duck, chicken, eggs, ham, fish, and seafood, but you will not add any grains, vegetables, fruits, nuts, or dairy to this meal. Keep the cooking as simple as possible. Avoid using store-bought sauces that can have lots of different ingredients and preservatives. Also avoid grilling because, as mentioned earlier, grilled (burned and browned) foods undergo glycation and are known to be carcinogenic.

Meats contain primarily protein and fat. The fat content of the meat triggers the satiety signal and therefore, generally, you cannot eat a huge amount of meat. You feel full, and you stop eating.

Digestion Time for Protein from Animal Sources

As with legumes, when meats are eaten by themselves, they get the entire stomach as well as the small intestine for their own digestion. The fiber and soluble carbohydrates from your breakfast and lunch have moved further down along the small intestine, so they do not interfere with digestion of meat. In addition, the next meal is going to be breakfast the next morning, so the meats have the entire night to be digested, absorbed, and eventually moved into the colon for stool formation.

Ideal Time for Dinner

About six hours after your midday meal, you will be ready for dinner. Having dinner between 6:00 and 7:00 p.m. is ideal. Eating too late at night is a habit created for a modern, city-based lifestyle. In agrarian societies, before the invention of electricity, people ate their dinners before sunset.

Ayurveda also recommends finishing dinner around dusk and not eating after the sun has set. This pattern of eating is more in tune with our biological rhythm, which is connected with the cycle of day and night. We wake up when the sun is coming up, feed ourselves and stay active during the daytime, and go to bed after the sun sets. This pattern of waking up, eating, and sleeping provides us with plenty of physical energy for day-to-day activities. And when this energy starts to decline, it is time for us to go to sleep.

However, the availability of electricity has brought artificial light into our life, and we fool ourselves into believing that because light is available, we can eat dinner as late as we want and then stay up to all hours of the night.

Breaking out of the cycle of natural light and spending our time in artificial light is known to cause stress, heart disease, ulcers, obesity, diabetes, depression, and accidents. Our body (particularly the pineal gland) makes melatonin in the darkness of night. This hormone is essential for health, sleep, and well-being. When we eat a heavy meal after sunset and remain awake in artificial light until late at night, our body stops making melatonin. A lack of melatonin affects our sleep, and a lack of sleep affects our overall well-being and causes the body to become sick with various illnesses.[80]

SIX-WEEK AND ONE-WEEK PROTOCOLS

The eight-week protocol described above might seem rather challenging and difficult to some people. Others might just breeze through it and come out feeling decades younger and pounds lighter, with many of their earlier health issues and discomforts struck off their list! For those who might want to simply dip their toes in the water first to see how it goes and maybe try entering a longer program later on, six-week and one-week versions are possible too.

SIX-WEEK AYURVEDIC RESET DIET PROTOCOL

A six-week protocol is simply two less weeks in the mixing/combining food stage of the eight-week protocol.

Week 1, Days 1 and 2: water only, water and herb tea only.

Week 1, Days 3, 4, 5, 6 and 7: one type of vegetable for a meal.

Week 2: same as week 1.

Week 3, Days 1 and 2: water only, water plus herb teas only.

Week 3, Days 3, 4, 5, 6 and 7: one type of fruit.

Week 4: same as week 3.

Week 5, Days 1 and 2: water only, water plus herb teas only.

Week 5, Days 3, 4, 5, 6 and 7: fruits and nuts for breakfast, vegetables and grains for lunch, legumes or meats for dinner.

Week 6: same as week 5.

ONE-WEEK AYURVEDIC RESET DIET PROTOCOL

In this abbreviated one-week version of the reset diet, the digestive system receives rest and training for extracting all nutrients from one type of fruit or vegetable that is eaten for a meal. A well-rested and rebooted digestive system is better able to handle food when a moderate and mindful normal eating pattern is resumed.

This simplified version will also give you an opportunity to restrict calories, eliminate toxic foods and toxic combinations from your meals, and clean up your gastrointestinal tract. Well worth doing—and if you ask me, some fasting and food isolating is better than none.

Day 1: fast on room temperature or warm water only.

Days 2, 3, and 4: eat only vegetables for breakfast, lunch, dinner, and snacks.

Days 5, 6, and 7: eat only fruits for breakfast, lunch, dinner, and snacks.

Ayurveda has a deep and keen insight into the health and disease states of the human body, and it understands the role and relationship of food in both. Our hunter-gatherer ancestors lived the lifestyle prescribed in Ayurveda: they were so in tune with nature that their food was also their medicine. Our modern foods are toxic and so is our modern lifestyle. The Ayurvedic reset diet gives you an opportunity to turn the clock back a little, reset and rebalance the body's ecosystem, and revitalize your prana. It helps you reestablish a healthy relationship with your food. The tools and techniques given in the three easy steps of the diet are a gift that you can use again and again for the rest of your life to maintain a great microbial ecosystem in your body that will keep many illnesses at bay.

Health and disease are part of the human experience. Both have a purpose and a role to play in our spiritual growth and progress. Our choices, actions, and ignorance can drive us toward the disease state. However, by practicing the techniques and simple steps given in the Ayurvedic reset diet, you can invest in your personal well-being and avail yourself of the opportunity to experience good health by rebooting and resetting your body.

7
Daily Living
Benefits, Challenges, and Next Steps

If you have made it this far, you should be seeing the benefits of the Ayurvedic reset diet. After completing two weeks of vegetables only and two weeks of fruits only, with two days of fasting at the beginning of each week, you will observe a reduction in weight and in the severity of gastrointestinal tract issues like yeast overgrowth, hernias, hemorrhoids, pains, stool irregularities, bloating, gas, acidity, and constipation. You will also experience more energy, alertness, and lightness in the body, along with a sharper and more focused mind, a cleaned, healed, and refreshed gastrointestinal tract, and a more immunologically healthy digestive system.

Some of my clients have lost anywhere from six to seventeen pounds. Other benefits besides weight loss and gastrointestinal tract wellness include a reduction in joint pain, fibromyalgia, depression, and a feeling of helplessness. And an added advantage is that your sense of accomplishment and pride in yourself increases because you have taken charge of your wellness, and you are doing something for your body that will have lasting impact on your overall health.

The ultimate success of the Ayurvedic reset diet and its ability to heal the gut is based on the following:

- Eating one food group at a time for weeks so that the digestive system is not burdened by the task of digesting huge amounts of many different types of foods at the same time
- Avoiding dairy, wheat, sugar, and processed foods
- Leaving a gap of six hours between two meals to clear out the earlier meal from the GI tract
- Eating in moderation

STAYING ON THE ISOLATION MEAL PLAN

You can continue the isolation meal plan laid out at the end of chapter 6 (pages 118–26)—fruits, vegetables, grains, and legumes or meats/eggs, eaten at different times of the day and not all together in one meal—for weeks at a time and could safely continue this way of eating as long as you prefer. Because the isolation meal plan gives you the chance to eat all the food groups, albeit only one food group at a time, you end up getting all the nutrients you need without any of the problems that arise from eating a combination of food groups that often lead to viruddha ahara. Some people begin to see the benefits of the plan, and they either continue this pattern of eating for longer periods of time or stop for a while and then resume it from time to time. Good habits, once learned, are hard to forget.

Between each week, maintain the two days of fasting: one day consuming water only and one day alternating between water and herbal tea. This is an essential practice. It gives the digestive system two days of rest and when you go back to eating food, your digestive system is better able to extract all the nutrients from it. Also, when food is withheld, the body turns its attention toward extracting energy from the reserves of glycogen and fat stored away in the body. Two days of abstaining from solid foods also comes with the advantage of restricting calorie intake. Calorie restriction is known to add longevity and facilitate improvement in general health.

GOING BACK TO REGULAR EATING

All that said, the biggest challenge to this might be boredom. People get tired of the same old, same old routine and they begin to look for change. So long as fruits, vegetables, legumes, grains, eggs, and meats along with modest amounts of fats are a part of your eating pattern, you will receive all the nutrients needed from your food. If one or a few of these items are omitted, and junk foods begin to take the place of the omitted food group, then the body will go back to its pre–reset diet state and the nutritional balance will suffer. One perceived advantage of going back to the regular, older pattern of eating is that people feel freer. They do not have to worry about eating out and eating in company. They can travel easily. And by eating a lot of different foods in one meal, they feel that they are having fun. But, all things considered, the food combining portion of the Ayurvedic reset diet is a sane way of eating that allows you the luxury of eating everything healthy in a way that the foods do not fight in your digestive system.

If you would rather go back to "regular eating" than stay on the meal plan, you can follow either one of the simpler plans below or go back to combined meals in which certain foods are reintroduced gradually.

SIMPLER MEAL PLAN FOR MEAT EATERS

If you include meat in your diet, eat eggs and nuts for breakfast. For lunch have two parts raw salad, one-part cooked vegetables, one-part whole grain and animal-based protein. At dinner, eat just vegetables and salads only or whole fruits only. Be sure to keep the six-hour gap between meals.

It is wise to minimize the use of red meat even if it happens to be organic. Focus more on poultry and seafood. Avoid processed and cured meats completely.

SIMPLER MEAL PLAN FOR VEGETARIANS

If you are a vegetarian, your breakfast can consist of nuts, seeds, and fruit smoothies. Lunch can be two parts salad, one-part cooked vegetables, and one-part whole grains and legumes. For dinner eat a large salad or just whole fruits.

For both styles of eating, fasting on water must be carried out at least one day per week. One day of fasting with water only and a second day with water and herbal teas alternating is still preferable and recommended. Also, be sure to follow the water-intake guidelines given on pages 104–5.

Reintroducing Fermented Foods

With the Ayurvedic reset diet, you have successfully shed the load of unnecessary germs from your gut and detoxified your whole body. Now is a good time to reintroduce healthy bacteria back into your gut. This can be done by including small amounts of fermented vegetables or beverages in your meal such as olives, dill pickles, sauerkraut, kimchi, and kombucha.[81] These contain a live probiotic mix of bacteria and yeast that are good for digestive system health. When consumed, these probiotics establish themselves amid the gut flora, and since the Ayurvedic reset diet has enabled us to flush out the unhealthy mix of gut flora from our system, these new strains of probiotics have an easier time colonizing the gut.

Reintroducing Dairy and Wheat

If you are not lactose intolerant or allergic to wheat, then as you begin eating combination meals, you can reintroduce these items. However, start gradually. Overloading your digestive system with foods that you have stayed away from is not a good idea. Starting with small quantities of these foods and consuming them infrequently is, however, a winning strategy.

Go for organic whole wheat, wheat germ, and germinated wheat and organic whole milk, cheese, butter, and yogurt. Even though whole milk has a full-fat content, this fat is better for you than artificially and chemically modified, low-fat dairy products. The trick is in consuming small quantities and not overeating anything, even if it is organic and wholesome.

FASTING AS A SUSTAINABLE METHOD OF WEIGHT MANAGEMENT, DISEASE PREVENTION, AND LONGEVITY

Getting back to a regular routine of eating everything in one meal is very tempting because it has been our lifelong habit. We never question the logic of a mixed meal, though we have incurred a heavy fine in the way of various illnesses that have come upon us from combining all the available industrially manufactured foods in one meal and the stress and tension of the modern, sedentary life we have gotten so used to.

To help with this situation, there are very convincing studies that support the point of view that calorie restriction is the way to go.[82] While you are on the Ayurvedic reset diet, each week is preceded by two days of fasting when you don't eat any solids and drink only water on one day and water alternating with herbal tea on the second day. If your "regular" combination meals give you 2,000 calories a day, say, you can shave off a total of 4,000 calories in one week just by fasting for two days. This practice can be continued going forward. Just simply make a decision to fast on water for one day and water alternating with herbal teas on the second day and allow this nectar of nature to flush and cleanse your entire system and help you lose weight. On the other five days, you can eat combination meals, but again, eating sensibly and in moderation are the keys to success.

The myth about fasting is that you will feel weak and have less energy for your daily tasks. That is what it actually is, a myth. Once you make a disciplined effort to make fasting into a routine, a habit, you will see that you actually begin to look forward to the fasting days because of the following reasons:

- You do not have to spend time cooking food or washing dishes and can use the extra time for other constructive activities and hobbies.

- Your entire body feels lighter, fresher, and cleaner after the fast.
- Your digestive system gets a chance to rest, rejuvenate, and recharge.
- Food tastes much better after the fast.
- Your digestion, absorption of nutrients, and elimination of wastes improves.
- Your overall health begins to improve.
- Your blood chemistry begins to improve, and cholesterol, diabetes, and digestive system disorders become manageable.
- Your general disposition, mood, energy level, and enthusiasm for life improves too because you are doing something creative, constructive, and solid for your own well-being.

Gandhi's Political Fasts

Mahatma Gandhi, the founding father of India, undertook fasting on seventeen occasions for a variety of reason. His first experiences of fasting were focused on health, then he progressed to spiritually motivated fasts, and ultimately even used fasting as a political tool. Whenever he undertook fasting with an agenda, he made national and international headlines. He had several different agendas for resisting the policies of the British rulers and he did so by using the principles and practice of nonviolence as well as fasting. He fasted on just water, and sometimes he would even abstain from that. His whole plan was to convey to the British that if they did not hear him and his people, then he would let go of food, let go of water, and simply die from starvation. Even with all his fasting, he was full of good cheer and good energy. Fasting often allowed him to work for longer hours with deeper concentration, and on his shorter fasts he could even keep up with his exercise routine.

After very heavy eating during celebrations or when you return home from traveling where the discipline of healthy eating is hard to maintain, it is a good idea to go back to the isolation meal plan for at least one week. You can follow the one-week Ayurvedic reset diet protocol described on page 127.

After this week, you can return gradually to your combined meal plan.

MOVING FORWARD

On thinking about the impact of modernization and industrialization making cheap industrial foods available to the masses, it is evident that the clock cannot be turned back. Our individual and collective past is out of reach. Our future is not yet born. All we have on hand is the present moment. But we can look back and learn about the life of our hunter-gatherer ancestors who lived on every continent of the earth before they were wiped out in genocides across the globe.

All the aborigines and native tribes were essentially tied to their place. Their identity, their foods, and their stories were also tied to their place. They walked about for spiritual quest, as a rite of passage or for food, but only within their own range, their own place. And in that place-bound existence, the natural order provided them knowledge about how to live and how to fend for themselves while living in sync with nature. They lived among their own kith and kin, and their place provided for all their needs.

Now, however, we are living in the Kali Yuga, the great age of mixing. We travel, intermarry, live in other countries, and eat food grown in other countries. This great mixing cannot be avoided or prevented anymore. It is as if nature and the great cycle of time are allowing it to happen. There is no point in fighting it, and there is no way this clock can ever be turned back.

Our salvation comes from doing the best we can in the circumstances that we find ourselves in. We are living in a modern, industrial and technological age. Our lives depend on electricity and fast transportation, and our smart phones and tablets travel with us wherever we go. There are very few people among us, if any at all, who would want to give up everything and go to the forest to start living a hunter-gatherer lifestyle. That leaves us with only one option: do the best we can in the moment we happen to be living. With this clarity, we can choose to lean toward organic, locally grown, and seasonal foods to the best of our ability and to use our resources wisely.

As I see it, our life is like our hand. A state of radiant well-being, the palm, is in the center, and it receives ongoing healing and support from the following five fingers:

1. Fasting and improving diet and nutrition for disease prevention
2. Spiritual practices and higher, positive aspirations for mental wellness
3. Healthy familial and social relationships for emotional wellness
4. Exercise in the form of walking, yoga, swimming, weight lifting, cycling, and so on for physical fitness
5. Healing modalities (modern medicine as well as all the other alternative systems from every culture and continent) for physical wellness

Engaging in just one or a few of these measures is not sufficient because such a partial, half-hearted engagement creates an imbalance in life and our life force begins to become diminished instead of shining radiantly. A hand is complete only with the presence and activity of all five fingers, and when even one finger is injured or missing, the hand suffers in functionality and appearance. Similarly, only when all of the above-mentioned disciplines are engaged does our life attain balance and radiance.

Taking better care of ourselves is a lifelong healing journey. It begins with a commitment to making significant lifestyle changes like learning to eat differently on the Ayurvedic reset diet. Making this commitment and sticking with it provides the necessary foundation on which the success of spiritual practices, relationships, physical discipline and exercise, and any or all medical/alternative-healing modalities depend. Just as the five fingers and the palm work together to do everything that we need the hand to do, our lifestyle practices and medical/alternative-healing modalities work together with our commitment to change to make radiant good health and well-being a true reality in our lives.

Namaste.
The radiant being within me greets the radiant being within you.

Notes

1. A good resource to learn more about the koshas is Harish Johari's *Chakras: Energy Centers of Transformation* (Rochester, Vt.: Destiny Books, 2000), 25–27.
2. William Li, *Eat to Beat Disease: The New Science of How the Body Can Heal Itself* (New York: Grand Central Publishing, 2019).
3. Samuel Hahnemann, *Organon of Medicine* (New Delhi, India: B. Jain Publishers, 2003), 282–83.
4. Ashkan Afshin et al., "Health Effects of Dietary Risks in 195 Countries, 1990–2017: A Systematic Analysis for the Global Burden of Disease Study 2017," *Lancet,* April 3, 2019.
5. Sarah Boseley, "Bad Diets Killing More People Globally than Tobacco, Study Finds," The Guardian (website), April 3, 2019.
6. These hymns can be found in the Valmiki Ramayana, Aranya Kanda, book 3, sarga 11.
7. Robert Lawlor, *Voices of the First Day: Awakening in the Aboriginal Dreamtime* (Rochester Vt.: Inner Traditions International, 1991), 1–11.
8. For more on the colonization and decimation of hunter-gatherer cultures see Jack Weatherford's *Indian Givers: How the Indians of the Americas Transformed the World* (New York: Crown Publishers, 1988); *Native Roots: How Indians Enriched America* (New York: Fawcett Books, 1991); and *Savages and Civilization: Who Will Survive?* (New York: Ballantine Books, 1994).
9. Samantha Olson, *How Three Meals a Day Became the Rule and Why We Should Be Eating Whenever We Get Hungry Instead*, Medical Daily (website), March 8, 2015.

10. Peter Brown, "Eat, Fast and Live Longer," Marishi Ayurveda Blogs (website), June 27, 2013.

11. S. Lock, "Eating Out Behavior in the U.S.—Statistics & Facts," Statista (website), March 1, 2018.

12. Robin Konie, *What's Really in a McDonald's Hamburger?* Thank Your Body (website), last updated February 7, 2020.

13. For more on the toxicity of food see Martin Teitel and Kimberly Wilson's *Genetically Engineered Foods: Changing the Nature of Nature; What You Need to Know to Protect Yourself, Your Family, and Our Planet* (Rochester, Vt.: Park Street Press, 2001).

14. Martin Teitel and Kimberly Wilson, *Genetically Engineered Foods: Changing the Nature of Nature* (Rochester, Vt.: Park Street Press, 2001).

15. "The Egg Industry" and "Chickens Used for Food," PETA (website).

16. "The Dairy Industry," PETA (website).

17. "Cow's Milk: A Cruel and Unhealthy Product," PETA (website).

18. "The Beef Industry," PETA (website); Jeremy Rifkin, *Beyond Beef: The Rise and Fall of the Cattle Culture* (New York: Penguin Books, 1992).

19. "Veal: A Byproduct of the Cruel Dairy Industry," PETA (website).

20. "The Pork Industry," PETA (website).

21. Kate Good, "Milk Life? How about Milk Destruction? The Shocking Truth about the Dairy Industry and the Environment," One Green Planet (website); Beth Gardiner, "How Growth in Dairy Is Affecting the Environment," *New York Times*, May 1, 2015.

22. Bryan Andres Murcia, "The Alarming Rate of Latin American Deforestation," Latin American Post (website), December 14, 2017.

23. For more on pasteurization see Ty Bollinger's "Why Pasteurized Milk Is Bad for Your Health," Truth about Cancer (website), September 27, 2016. For more on the microbial population of milk see Lisa Quigley et al.'s "The Complex Microbiota of Raw Milk," *FEMS Microbiology Reviews* 37, no. 5 (September 2013): 664–98.

24. Jamie Ducharme, "Why Whole Fat Milk and Yogurt Are Healthier Than You Think," TIME (website), September 2018; Markham Heid, "Why Full-Fat Dairy May Be Healthier Than Low Fat," TIME (website), March 5, 2015.

25. "Lactose Intolerance: Overview," NCBI (website), last updated November 29, 2018.

26. "Health Concerns about Dairy," Physicians Committee for Responsible Medicine (website).

27. D. Feskanich, et al., "Milk, Dietary Calcium, and Bone Fractures in Women: A 12-Year Prospective Study," *American Journal of Public Health* 87, no. 6 (June 1997): 992–97, NCBI (website).

28. T. Colin Campbell, "The Mystique of Protein and Its Implications," Center for Nutrition Studies (website), last updated January 3, 2019; Francis Vergunst and Julian Savulescu, "Five Ways the Meat on Your Plate Is Killing the Planet," Conversation (website), April 26, 2017.

29. Thibault Fiolet, et al., "Consumption of Ultra-Processed Foods and Cancer Risk: A Result from NutriNet-Santé Prospective Cohort," *British Medical Journal*, 360, no. k322 (2018), BMJ (website).

30. "Can Diet Influence the Onset of Early Puberty?" DrCarney (website), August 13, 2015.

31. For a good resource on the benefits of plant-based foods visit the Plantrician Project website.

32. Sandip T. Gaikwad, et al., "Principles of Fasting in Ayurveda," *International Journal of Science, Environment and Technology* 6, no. 1 (2017): 787–92; Shripathi Adiga and Ramya S. Adiga, "Apprehending and Applauding the Therapeutic Importance of Fasting in Ayurveda," *Journal of Nutrition, Fasting and Health* 4, no. 1 (2016): 48–52.

33. Yu-Jie Zhang, et al., "Impact of Gut Bacteria on Human Health and Diseases," *International Journal of Molecular Sciences* 16, no. 4 (April 2015): 7493–519; Eamonn Quigley, "Gut Bacteria in Health and Disease," *Gastroenterology & Hepatology* 9, no. 9 (September 2013): 560–69.

34. Masaru Emoto, *The Hidden Messages in Water* (New York: Atria Books, 2001).

35. For more science on the memory and vibrations of water see the following resources: Masaru Emoto, *The Secret Life of Water* (New York: Atria Books, 2005); Bill Gray, *Homeopathy: Science or Myth?* (Berkeley, Calif.: North Atlantic Books, 2000); Won H. Kim, "3D Wave Explains 'Water Memory'," *Fluid Mechanics: Open Access* 2, no. 2 (2015); John Stuart Reid, "New Water Memory Research May Lead to Better Understanding of Homeopathic Medicine," GreenMedinfo (website), August 2, 2018; Shui-Yin Lo et al., "Physical Properties of Water with I_E Structures," *Modern Physics Letters B* 10, no. 19 (1996): 921–30; Paolo Bellavite and Andrea Signorini, *The Emerging Science of Homeopathy: Complexity, Biodynamics, and Nanopharmacology* (Berkeley, Calif.: North Atlantic Books, 2002), 258–89; Shui-Yin Lo and Benjamin Bonavida, eds., *Physical, Chemical,*

and Biological Properties of Stable Water (I_E™) Clusters: Proceedings of the First International Symposium (Singapore: World Scientific Publishing Company, 1998).

36. For more on the science of Homeopathy see George Vithoulkas's *A New Model for Health and Disease* (Northern Sporades, Greece: International Academy of Classical Homeopathy, 1991); *Homeopathy: Medicine for the New Millennium* (Northern Sporades, Greece: International Academy of Classical Homeopathy, 1985); and *The Science of Homeopathy* (New Delhi, India: B. Jain Publishers, 1998).

37. "Water Distribution on Earth," Wikipedia (website).

38. Jane E. Stevens, "Oral Ecology," MIT Technology Review (website), January 1, 1997.

39. For more on fasting and glycogen see Valter D. Longo and Mark P. Mattson, "Fasting: Molecular Mechanisms and Clinical Applications," *Cellular Metabolism* 19, no. 2 (February 4, 2014): 181–92; Michele D. Moore, "Fasting Can Heal the Human Organism of Disease and Reverse the Ageing Process," *JOJ Dermatology and Cosmetics* 2, no. 2 (2019): 555581.

40. "The Nobel Prize in Physiology or Medicine 2016/Summary," Nobel Prize (website), May 15, 2020; Dara Mohammadi, "2016 Nobel Prize in Medicine Goes to Japanese Scientist," *Lancet, World Report* 388, no. 10054 (October 15, 2016): 1870.

41. Keki R. Sidhwa, "What Are the Effects of Fasting?" British Institute of Osteopathy (website), August 2007.

42. Gary Greenberg, "'Smart' Vacation Offers Water Fast," *Life Extension* (January–February 2019): 37–40.

43. Mukund Sabnis, "Viruddha Ahara: A Critical View," *Ayu* 33, no. 3 (July–Sept. 2012): 332–36, NCBI (website).

44. Anne Waugh and Allison Grant, *Ross and Wilson Anatomy and Physiology in Health and Illness*, 9th ed. (London: Churchill Livingstone, 2001), 293–303.

45. Waugh and Grant, *Ross and Wilson,* 314–15.

46. Jennifer Huizen, "Soluble and Insoluble Fiber: What Is the Difference?" Medical News Today (website), 2017.

47. Alice Park, "Want to Prevent Deadly Diseases? Eat More Fiber," *TIME* (February 18–25, 2019): 110.

48. Waugh and Grant, *Ross and Wilson,* 293–303, 316–17.

49. Waugh and Grant, *Ross and Wilson,* 302.

50. Waugh and Grant, *Ross and Wilson,* 317–18.

51. Jamie Ducharme, "Why Whole Fat Milk and Yogurt Are Healthier Than You Think," TIME (website), September 2018; Markham Heid, "Why Full-Fat Dairy May Be Healthier Than Low Fat," TIME (website), March 5, 2015.

52. "Butter Is Alright but Margarine Just Might Kill You," *Telegraph,* National Post (website), August 2015.

53. She-Chung Wu and Gow Chin Yen, "Effect of Cooking Oil Fumes on the Genotoxicity and Oxidative Stress in Human Lung Carcinoma (A-549) Cells," *Toxicology In Vitro* 18, no. 5 (October 2004): 571–80; E. Vladykovaskaya, et al., "Lipid Peroxidation Product 4-Hydroxy Trans-2-Nonenal Causes Endothelial Reticulum Stress," *Journal of Biological Chemistry* 287, no. 14 (March, 30, 2012): 11398–409; Huiqin Zhong and Huiyong Yin, "Role of Lipid Peroxidation Derived 4-Hydroxynonenal (4-HNE) in Cancer: Focusing on Mitochondria," *Redox Biology* 4, no. 193–99 (April 2015); "The Truth about Fats: The Good, the Bad and the In-Between," Harvard Health Publishing (website), 2015; Robin Madell and Rachel Nall, "Good Fats, Bad Fats and Heart Disease," Healthline (website), 2018; Yangbo Sun et al., "Association of Fried Food Consumption with all Cause, Cardiovascular, and Cancer Mortality: Prospective Cohort Study," *British Medical Journal* (online) 364 (January 23, 2019).

54. "Nutrients Lost during Cooking," TNAU Agritech Portal (website).

55. William E. Kraus et al., "2 Years of Calorie Restriction and Cardiometabolic Risk (CALERIE): Exploratory Outcomes of a Multicentre, Phase 2, Randomised Controlled Trial," *Lancet* 7, no. 9 (September 1, 2019): 673–83.

56. Kevin D. Hall et al., "Ultra-Processed Diets Cause Excess Calorie Intake and Weight Gain: An Inpatient Randomized Controlled Trial of *Ad Libitum* Food Intake," *Cell Metabolism* 30, no. 1 (July 2, 2019): 67–77.

57. Farokh J. Master, *Healing Cancer: A Homeopathic Approach,* vol. 1 (New Delhi, India: B. Jain Publishers, 2019), 98–102.

58. Some good references on growing your own container garden are Dixie Sandborn's "Container Gardening for Growing Food" (from Michigan State University MSU Extension's website) and "Growing Vegetables in Containers" (from the University of Florida Gardening Solutions' website).

59. "The Honey Industry," PETA (website).

60. Jamie Ducharme, "The Rise of Healthier Proteins," *TIME* (January 28, 2019): 53–55.

61. Ducharme, "The Rise of Healthier Proteins," 53–55.

62. "Seasonal Produce Guide," SNAP-Ed Connection (website).

63. R. Eberhard, et al., "Phosphate Additives in Foods: A Health Risk," *Deutsches Ärzteblatt International* 109, no. 4 (January 2012): 49–55; Benjamin P. Best, "Cryoprotectant Toxicity: Facts, Issues, and Questions," *Rejuvenation Research* 18, no. 5 (October 1, 2015): 422–36.

64. "Meat Products with High Levels of Extenders and Fillers," Food and Agriculture Organization of the United States (website).

65. Nicole M. Avena, Pedro Rada, and Bartley G. Hoebel, "Evidence for Sugar Addiction: Behavioral and Neurochemical Effects of Intermittent, Excessive Sugar Intake," *Neuroscience and Biobehavioral Reviews* 32, no. 1 (2008): 20–39.

66. Christopher Kilham, *The Five Tibetans: Five Dynamic Exercises for Health, Energy, and Personal Power* (Rochester, Vt.: Healing Arts Press, 1994).

67. Anne Tergesen, "The Best Exercises for Your 50s, 60s, 70s—and Beyond," Wall Street Journal (website), April 19, 2019.

68. Martin M. Grajower and Benjamin D. Horne, "Clinical Management of Intermittent Fasting in Patients with Diabetes Mellitus," *Nutrients* 11, no. 4 (April 18, 2019): 873; Suleiman Furmli et al., "Therapeutic Use of Intermittent Fasting for People with Type 2 Diabetes as an Alternative to Insulin," *British Medical Journal* Case Reports 2018 (October 9, 2018).

69. Otilia Bobis, et al., "Honey and Diabetes: The Importance of Natural Simple Sugars in Diet for Preventing and Treating Different Types of Diabetes," OxiMed & Cellular Longevity (website) vol. 2018, article 4757893.

70. David Hoffman, *Medical Herbalism: The Science Principles and Practices of Herbal Medicine* (Rochester Vt.: Healing Arts Press, 2003), 258–315, 571; Lizzie Streit, "9 Teas That Can Improve Digestion," Healthline (website), August 14, 2019; "Herbs & the Digestive System," Traditional Medicinals (website), October 26, 2016.

71. Ted Kallmyer, "Caffeine Withdrawal Symptoms: Top Fifteen," Caffeine Informer (website), last updated April 30, 2020.

72. Erica Cirino, "What Happens When You Drink on an Empty Stomach?" Healthline (website), October 23, 2018.

73. Katherine Watson, "Enema Administration," Healthline (website), January 24, 2017.

74. Christopher Vasey, *The Detox Mono Diet: The Miracle Grape Cure and Other Cleansing Diets* (Rochester, Vt.: Healing Arts Press, 1995), 132–33.

75. See Wu, "Effect of Cooking Oil Fumes"; Vladykovaskaya, "Lipid Peroxidation"; and Zhong, "Role of Lipid Peroxidation" in note 49.
76. "Water Intake Calculator" Aqua4Balance (website).
77. Vasey, *Detox Mono Diet*.
78. "How Much Time Your Body Takes to Digest These Foods," Times Food (website), November 16, 2018.
79. "Legumes and Nutrition" and "Legumes and Fiber," Grains & Legumes Nutrition Council (website).
80. "The Health Risks of Shift Work," *Web*MD (website).
81. "Discover the Digestive Benefits of Fermented Foods," Health & Nutrition Letter (Tufts University website), January 29, 2014; Kelly Bilodeau, "Fermented Foods for Better Gut Health," Harvard Health Publishing (website), May 16, 2018.
82. Many articles on calorie restriction (117+ available to date) can be found on the Life Extension website.

Index